UN_plug the Christmas machine_

UNplug

Jo Robinson and
Jean Coppock Staeheli

the Christmas machine

✳ A complete guide to putting
love and joy back into the season

REVISED EDITION

Quill
WILLIAM MORROW
New York

It is the policy of William Morrow and Company, Inc., and its imprints and affiliates, recognizing the importance of preserving what has been written, to print the books we publish on acid-free paper, and we exert our best efforts to that end.

Library of Congress Cataloging-in-Publication Data

Robinson, Jo, 1947–
    Unplug the Christmas machine : a complete guide to putting love and joy back into the season / Jo Robinson & Jean Coppock Staeheli
        p.   cm.
    ISBN 0-688-10961-6
    1. Christmas. 2. Simplicity. 3. Christmas decorations.
    4. Christmas—United States.   I. Staeheli, Jean Coppock.
    II. Title.
    GT4985.R62   1991b
    394.2′68282—dc20   91-14258
                                                                                              CIP

Printed in the United States of America

    5 6 7 8 9 10

BOOK DESIGN BY BINNS & LUBIN / BETTY BINNS

*   We dedicate this book to
all the people who have shared their
Christmas stories with us.

OTHER BOOKS CO-AUTHORED BY JO ROBINSON

Full House (Little, Brown & Co., 1986)

Getting the Love You Want (Henry Holt, 1989)

The Emotional Incest Syndrome (Bantam, 1990)

※

———

CONTENTS

※

※

※

※

Contents
✳

People often ask us whether Christmas has changed for the better since the first edition of this book was published in 1982. The answer is both yes and no.

Yes, we see more people making conscious choices during the holiday season. The month of December can be like an overfilled Christmas stocking, bursting with beautifully wrapped concerts, parties, family re-unions, shopping expeditions, craft and baking projects, and special events. More families are sitting down together in early November and setting priorities. As a result, they are creating rich celebrations that suit their circumstances and reflect their values, but don't feel hectic and out of control.

We see a greater number of women being more relaxed about holiday preparations. The woman who tells her friend that, this year, she "did it all" is more likely to evoke concern than admiration from her listener. Women are freer to let go of the internal injunction that they have to be all things to all people. Not surprisingly, this means that their husbands are showing more interest in the holiday. When women let go of some of the control of the celebration, men begin to fill in the vacuum. In many households across the country, Christmas is truly becoming a family affair.

We have talked with many people who are accepting the fact that family demographics have changed. The Perfect Family at Christmas—the one with a loving mom and dad, two biological children, and a full complement of cousins, aunts, uncles, and adoring grandparents—is now a rarity. A quite different cast of characters gathers around the Christmas tree in the 1990s. In one household, an only child might be unwrapping a mound of gifts while her parents and grandparents watch in adoration. Across the street, a single mother might be getting ready to drive her two children to their father's house for another round of gift opening. Next door, the house might be teeming with children—two from the mother's previous marriage, two from the father's previous marriage, a brand-new baby from the new marriage, and an assortment of cousins.

A block away, two gay men might may be listening to Christmas carols on the CD player as they wish each other a Merry Christmas. And across town, two unrelated families might be joining forces to make up for the fact that all their relatives live in different parts of the country. And these quite different family groupings are beginning to feel okay.

Another change we've observed is that the food on the Christmas table is likely to be less rich, less elaborate, and less abundant than it was nine years ago, and people are discovering that this trend toward moderation does not detract from their enjoyment. What does detract is drinking too much. We hear people say that getting drunk on eggnog is more an indication of a serious problem, or, at least, a violation of good taste, than a seasonal exhibition of good spirits.

People used to laugh when we asked them whether or not they took good care of themselves during the holiday season. Healthy habits and seasonal celebrating were incompatible, or so it seemed. Now people take our "healthy life-style" question seriously. They tell us that even if they don't take care of themselves during the holiday season, they believe they should.

Some aspects of Christmas have been slow to change, however. As a nation, we are still spending a lot of money to wish each other a Merry Christmas. In fact, economists now estimate we are spending considerably more than the twenty billion dollars that we were spending in 1982. Then, as now, gift giving and holiday spending habits are the most entrenched. Despite the many changes people are making each December, they still feel as if they are inexorably swept up into the engine of the Christmas Machine.

The Christmas Machine has this power over us because it knows how to woo us; it speaks to the deepest, profoundest, and most sacred desires of the human heart. If it appeared as a monster, we would rise up and stop it. But the commercial messages of Christmas appear as promises that bring tears to our eyes. Look at the bounty we are promised by the December magazines and the glowing Christmas commercials:

Our families will be together and be happy.
Our children will be well-behaved and grateful.
Our wives will be beautiful and nurturing.
Our husbands will be kind, generous, and appreciative.

We will have enough money.
We will have enough time.
We will have fun.
We will be warm.
We will be safe.
We will be truly loved.

No wonder we stop, we listen, and we want to believe. The problem comes when we buy into the notion that what we long for can be procured by the buying and selling of goods. Okay. We know it's nonsensical to expect that buying a new phone as a gift for a parent or a video camera to capture the excitement of Christmas morning or a new pair of designer jeans for a son or daughter will transform our lives. But it's easy to be persuaded by the artistry of the commercials, with their exquisite photography and their beautiful music. Sometimes, somehow, an association does get made with the product, and we believe that if we buy and receive more Christmas presents our inner lives will be fuller, and we will finally be safe in the world.

Another reason we've been slow to Unplug the Christmas Machine is that the Machine has a human face. It's the face of the nice lady who owns the bookshop you love to browse in. It's the department store executive who is responsible for his store's seasonal ad campaign and who also has two kids at home who are excited about Christmas. It's the clerk in the gift shop who has been arranging ornaments, pomander balls, and candles on the shop shelves since the end of October. It's your neighbor who is grateful for his seasonal job at a local department store. These people are the Machine and they are also caught in the Machine, wishing Christmas could be simpler and more joyful.

The Machine affects us all, each of us differently. We are susceptible to its rules and injunctions, depending on our vulnerability. The working mother who lives day in and day out with the nagging feeling that she should be doing more for her children is an easy target. When she sees an ad that tells her she can ensure her daughter's happy memories by buying a hundred-dollar doll, she is extraordinarily open to the suggestion. The husband whose self-esteem is fragile because he's just been passed over for a promotion may find himself going into debt to buy diamond earrings for his wife as a testimony to his ability to provide.

The child who is unsure of his parent's love may generate a long gift list because he wants proof his folks are paying attention, that they care. After Christmas, this same child may shovel his new presents into his room and wonder why he still didn't get what he really wanted.

And *that*, we've discovered, is the key to Unplugging the Machine —knowing what it is that you really want. People who take the time to identify their longings, and are realistic about which of those longings can be satisfied by Christmas, can then go on to create a holiday that gives them great joy and satisfaction. We hope that what you learn in the following pages will help you do this. In this revised edition we have gathered together the best of the insights and suggestions from twelve years of talking to people about Christmas and put them into a package designed to help you resolve your unique holiday problems or enrich an already enjoyable celebration.

Jo Robinson and Jean Staeheli

P.S. This year, you can not only enrich your own celebration, you can help the members of your church, school, parents' group, business, or other organization create a more enjoyable, less stressful holiday season by holding an Unplug the Christmas Machine Workshop. This four-hour workshop has already been given by over a thousand diverse organizations in the United States and Canada. We have written a *Leader's Guide* which contains everything you need to conduct a successsful workshop. It is available from William Morrow and Company for $20.00 or you can order it from your local bookstore. (See the order form on page 195.)

The Christmas Pledge

✳

Believing in the true spirit of Christmas,
I commit myself to

✳

Remember those people who truly
need my gifts

✳

Express my love in more direct ways than gifts

✳

Examine my holiday activities in the light
of my deepest values

✳

Be a peacemaker within my circle of
family and friends

✳

Rededicate myself to my spiritual growth

In the many years we've spent talking to people about Christmas, we've catalogued a lot of common problems people have during the holiday season. Many people feel pressured by all the work involved in orchestrating the family celebration. Many people are worried about holiday bills. Some people are worried about how to survive Christmas after a recent loss, such as a divorce, death in the family, or layoff from a job. And others are troubled by the fact that they are childless or single or estranged from their families and wonder how they can piece together a memorable celebration.

But the one concern that unites virtually all the people we've talked to is a yearning for a simpler, less commercial, more soul-satisfying celebration. There is a universal wish to end the year with a festival of renewal that rekindles our faith, brings us closer to the people we care about, and brings light and laughter to the dark days of winter. We want to ward off the commercial excesses of the season and create an authentic, joyful celebration in tune with our unique needs and desires.

But is this possible? We've noticed that many people come to our workshops with an air of resignation. Although they're unhappy about holiday commercialism—"Why do the ads have to start so early?" "Why is there so much pressure to buy, buy, buy?"—they don't have much faith in their ability to unplug the Christmas Machine. And although they freely admit to feeling hassled in those hectic weeks leading up to Christmas and then let down by the celebration itself, they aren't convinced they can make any significant changes. That's the way Christmas is for adults: stressful and ultimately disappointing. The most they dare hope for from us is a few tips on coping with holiday stress, and perhaps some answers to a few specific problems.

By the end of a workshop, however, most people are filled with enthusiasm and have a newfound optimism about their ability to transform the celebration. They see that Christmas can be a rewarding, spiritual—even relaxing—time of year, and they are determined to make this happen. Part of this turnaround can be traced to the insights they

※

*Chapter
one*

___

**"A
CHRISTMAS
CAROL"
REVISITED**

※

※

※

※

15

have gained in completing the key workshop exercises. In the space of four hours, they've had a chance to pinpoint what they like and don't like about their current celebrations, clarify their values, get in touch with their fantasies, and create a simple plan to move toward a more satisfying celebration. (You will find all of these exercises in this book.)

But people tell us that another part of the workshop that helps them a great deal is our ten-minute "mini-lecture" on the history of the Christmas Machine. When they have a better sense of the many subtle ways that commercialism has altered Christmas, they can see why the modern celebration seems so flat and uninspiring. And for the first time, they get a glimpse of some specific ways they can add more warmth and vitality to their own celebrations.

To find out what the old-fashioned Christmas was really like, the two of us spent several days sequestered in the library. Like most people today, we grew up in a time when Christmas was heavily commercialized, so our vision of Christmas Past was a blurry pastiche of Currier and Ives prints and heart-tugging scenes from *The Little House on the Prairie*.

We began to fill in some of the gaps in our knowledge when we cranked our way through reels of microfilm of December newspapers from the late 1800s. During this period of our country's history, we saw little evidence of the Christmas Machine. There were only a few holiday ads, most of them devoted to children's toys. The one or two ads targeted at adults displayed simple gifts called "holiday notions." If our grandparents and great-grandparents exchanged presents at all, they probably gave gifts on the order of pipe tobacco, books, a packet of pins, or hand-embroidered handkerchiefs.

This simpler, less commercial Christmas is reflected in Christmas literature from the 1800s. Think for a moment about the heartwarming Christmas dinner in Bob Cratchit's house in Dickens's "Christmas Carol." Remember the warm welcome when daughter Martha walked in the door, glad to be home for the festive meal? Remember the young Cratchit children dancing around the table, unable to contain their enthusiasm over the aroma of the sage and onion stuffing? Remember Tiny Tim beating on the table with the handle of his knife in exultation over the Christmas goose?

The only thing missing from this animated scene was any evidence of gifts. Although Tiny Tim may have found some trinkets in his stocking on Christmas morning, it is unlikely there would have been any gifts for the older children or for Bob and Mrs. Cratchit. In all but the wealthy families in Victorian England, gifts were reserved for the very young. The adults regarded Christmas as a time to feast, sing, and play riotous games. This is why Scrooge bah-humbugged his way through the holiday: There was little way for him to profit from the celebration.

The fact that gift giving was of minor importance for adults in the nineteenth century had a profound effect on the celebration. First of all, holiday preparations could be less elaborate. A pioneer homemaker in Nebraska didn't have to spend weeks shopping for gifts, wrapping them, and then standing in long lines at the post office. Nor did she have the anxiety of wondering if she had chosen just the right gift for all the adults on her list. Instead, she could concentrate her energy on the baking and decorating and making a few gifts for the children.

Second, the absence of an elaborate gift-giving tradition meant that the holiday could stay anchored in its appropriate season. There was no need for our great-grandmothers to make gifts in the heat of July so their adult sisters and brothers could have an abundance of gifts on Christmas morning. They could sew the linsey-woolsey dresses for their daughters and the dress shirts for their sons in the cool of December.

Furthermore, our ancestors didn't have to steel themselves against a barrage of premature holiday advertising. They could glory in the golds and browns of fall before seeing any hint of the reds and greens of Christmas. When they began to prepare for the holiday around mid-December, their actions felt in sync with the seasons. For our ancestors, the celebration was truly a winter festival.

Finally, unlike today, the old-fashioned Christmas didn't come to a screeching halt once the gifts were opened. For adults, the morning of December 25 heralded the *beginning* of the celebration, not the end. Once the children had emptied their stockings and the adults had exclaimed over their simple, "holiday notions," everyone could look forward to a church service followed by days of visiting, family games, and joyous Christmas dances. The Twelve Days of Christmas could officially begin.

Here's a description of a Christmas party, from an article in the December 1895 issue of *Good Housekeeping*, to which our ancestors might have been invited in those festive days between Christmas and New Year's.

*Each Christmas we'd converge on a long, wide, cheerful farm house
kitchen and play games like "wade the swamp," "keep post office," "pick
grapes," "measure tape," and "hiss cat."*

*Sometimes we danced, with the fiddlers perched high on kitchen tables.
There was no mincing along on one's toes with every stop "just so.". . .
We "swung our pardners" as partners are not often swung, sometime
lifting them quite off their feet. We danced to the good old tunes of "Dan
Tucker" and "Money-musk" and we kept it up until broad day-light in the
morning.*

*There was nothing formal about these affairs. Nothing graceful, nothing
"put-on," nothing refined, but those who attended them were genuinely
and unaffectedly happy and Christmas meant much to them.*

This high-spirited celebration was still in evidence in this country
at the turn of the century, but as time went on, there began to appear
more and more signs of commercialism. This was apparent to us as we
continued our search through the microfilms. In the newspapers from
the first decade of this century, for example, we began to see an increasing
number of holiday ads targeted at adults, and the gifts that were advertised
were becoming more extravagant. Ads promoting jewelry for women and
waistcoats for men now appeared alongside the ads for dolls and trains
for children. To a large degree, this reflected a general trend in the
United States toward a consumer economy. Mass production was making
goods readily available, and the population as a whole was becoming
more affluent. However, holiday sales merited special consideration. In
our research we came across a 1906 tradebook for retailers entitled *Merchant's Record and Show Window* which contained complete instructions
for creating a "perfected holiday advertising machinery running full
blast." The Christmas Machine was quickly gathering steam.

As we scanned the 1918 and 1919 newspapers, we noticed another
upsurge in holiday advertising. Now the ads were appearing a full month
before Christmas, and they were more aggressive in tone. Retailers were
no longer content to modestly describe the worthiness of their goods;
they were launching a frontal assault on the psyche of the shopper. For
example, we found this ad that appeared in *The New York Times* on
December 15, 1919: "Don't give your family and friends frivolous gifts
that are sure to disappoint, buy them worthy gifts that will let them
know how much you care." Another ad from the same period features
a sketch of a disdainful looking man with a cigarette hanging out of his

mouth. The ad copy advises women that their husbands will be highly critical of their offerings unless they come from a certain elegant men's store. A woman who was accustomed to slipping a necktie or some tobacco into Papa's stocking was being issued a blunt warning that she had better spend more money if she valued domestic tranquillity.

It is no accident that this more militant holiday advertising coincided with the end of World War I. At that time, there were fears that the unprecedented boom times of World War I were going to be followed by a stagnant economy. So to make up for the dwindling war contracts, advertisers turned their newly developed "science of persuasion" into an all-out campaign to stimulate consumer spending. Christmas gift giving was a prime target. After all, the idea of generosity was firmly embedded in the celebration; all the advertisers had to do was capitalize on it.

The campaign succeeded beyond anyone's wildest dreams. Department store inventories rose more than 50 percent between 1919 and 1920. By 1923, the amount of money that American consumers were spending on surplus consumption (including but not limited to Christmas) equaled the amount of money that had been coming into the nation's coffers during the last years of World War I. Sadly, there appears to be some truth to the adage that the American economy is fueled by war and Christmas.

In all fairness, it must be said that the engineers of the Christmas Machine found a ready and willing audience for their wares. For the most part, people were delighted to give their families the opulent celebrations that were once the province of the rich. It seemed like a step in the direction of progress to give their children bicycles and electric trains instead of doughnuts and rag dolls. Since people had no way of knowing how commercialization would impoverish the holiday, they had no reason to resist it.

From that point on, the Christmas Machine lurched into high gear. Stores began offering "Special Liberal Xmas Credit" for shoppers whose Yuletide enthusiasm outstripped their available cash. Advertisers discovered that the amount of money people spent was influenced more by the length of the advertising campaign than the length of people's gift lists, so they began their promotions earlier and earlier each year. From the first preholiday sale in October to the last postholiday clearance in mid-January, people were deluged with advertising. Soon, we were spending billions of dollars a year to wish each other a "Merry Little Christmas," as retail stores reaped from 25 to 50 percent of their annual profits from holiday sales.

Little has changed in recent decades except for the fact that the Christmas Machine has become more elegant and refined; today's sophisticated audience demands a more genteel approach. Advertisers of the 1990s lure us into the better stores not with bombastic ads but with live woodwind quartets playing French Christmas carols. Savvy store decorators pack away the glitz and the tinsel in favor of live poinsettias and cascades of twinkling white lights. And we are invited into shopping malls whose façades are festooned with Victorian Christmas ornaments and ornate signs proclaiming the "Dickens's Christmas Spirit." In the lush display we are lulled into forgetting that the true Christmas spirit of Dickens had to do with family traditions, the love of humanity, and compassion for the poor—not the marketing needs of a consumer economy.

To see in sharp contrast how Christmas of today differs from Christmas of a hundred fifty years ago, imagine for a moment that Dickens were writing "A Christmas Carol" today. Change the setting of his classic cautionary tale from the sooty streets of Victorian London to the smoggy suburbs of Los Angeles. Now update the main characters. Ebenezer Scrooge is now the proud owner of a shopping mall. Unlike his nineteenth-century counterpart, he is enamored with Christmas because every ring of the cash register adds to his fourth-quarter profits. Hear him whistle "Deck the Halls" as he supervises the early October decorating of the mall. Watch him chortle as he tallies up each day's receipts. See him gather his clerks for an early-morning motivational meeting, admonishing them to wish all the customers a cheery "Merry Christmas."

Now summon poor, beleaguered Bob Cratchit, a minor accountant at Scrooge Enterprises, who, like many men today, has a cynical attitude toward Christmas. See him fret on the way to work, "How in the world am I going to afford Air Jordans for Tiny Tim, a portable CD player for Peter, Guess? jeans for Martha, and a leather flight jacket for Belinda? And now Mrs. Cratchit tells me she wants a two-hundred-dollar Dooney & Bourke handbag. Thank goodness they've just raised the limit on my Visa card." Hear him grouse to the guys at lunch, "Christmas has gotten so commercial! I saw the first holiday ads in October this year! I don't think I'll get through December without a major depression."

See Bob drive up to his bungalow to be greeted by a harried Mrs.

Cratchit: "Honey, I've been wrapping the last gifts to send to your mother in New York, but I've run out of ribbon. Could you dash over to the mall for some wrapping supplies? If I stay up tonight to finish the wrapping, I can mail the presents during my lunch break tomorrow—unless, of course, you want me to wait another day and send them Federal Express." Watch Bob slink back to the car, muttering under his breath. "The last thing I need to do right now is fight the bumper-to-bumper holiday traffic and the crowds at the mall. The only good thing about Christmas is the football games. Bah! Humbug!"

It's no wonder that so many people feel disappointed by Christmas. It's not that they don't like the holiday, it's that they don't like what's *happened* to it. People tell us that Christmas has become increasingly impersonal, frenetic, costly, and empty of meaning. Busy women feel pressured to put on a year-end extravaganza and are given the hidden message that their families' happines depends on their nonstop performance. Men are assigned only a minor role in the festivities, yet are criticized for their lack of enthusiasm. And children are programmed to believe that what they really want for Christmas are dozens of brand-name toys, and are rarely given the time and attention that would satisfy their unspoken needs.

But Christmas doesn't have to be this way. What we have discovered in the past ten years is that people can write their own versions of the "Christmas Carol," keeping all the love and joy of the Cratchit family Christmas, but tailoring it to their modern circumstances. The stories will be different for each household, but there will be a common theme uniting them all. As we were preparing this second edition, we thumbed through our files and came across the following quotation from a December 1913 issue of *Good Housekeeping*. We were struck anew by the truth of its sentiments. Although Christmas is always changing, the key elements of the celebration endure:

> . . . while winter is white and cold and human hearts are warm, Christmas must continue to be the universal festival of peace and good will, the sacred season of love, the holiday of kindness. Its innovations will but celebrate new modes of happiness and new ways of being kind.

We hope that by reading this book you will discover some "new modes of happiness."

※

Chapter

two

———

WOMEN: THE CHRISTMAS MAGICIANS

※

※

※

※

When we listen to people talk about Christmas, often the first thing they mention is holiday commercialism. "Why do the stores have to decorate so early?" "Why do the ads have to start in October?" But as the conversation becomes more intimate, they begin talking about the way their own celebrations have gotten out of hand: "Why does it take me four weeks to get ready for Christmas?" "Why is my family so hung up on gifts?" At times it seems like they, too, are caught up in the Christmas Machine and are making choices based on habit and external pressure, not their own needs and values.

Women tend to feel this disappointment most acutely because they are the Christmas Magicians, responsible for transforming their families' everyday lives into a beautiful festival. No matter how busy they are, they bear the burden of pulling a magical celebration out of the hat year after year. Like their mothers before them, they are the planners, the shoppers, the decorators, the gift-wrappers, the bakers, the hostesses, and the housecleaners. If the celebration doesn't feel right—if it seems too hectic, or superficial, or if family problems erupt—then they feel that they are to blame.

Women have always played this central role in the celebration. Christmas is not only a religious holiday but a celebration of hearth and home, and it makes sense that women should take the lead. But in this century, Christmas has become more elaborate, and women's lives have become more complex. Today's Mrs. Cratchit leads a busy life outside the home and is likely to be found stirring up the plum pudding late at night. She not only buys and wraps the gifts, she may hold down an outside job to pay for them as well. If she also happens to be a single parent, then she must be a very skillful Christmas Magician indeed.

Examining the role that women play at Christmas is a key part of our workshops. The fact that most women have mixed feelings about the holiday is evident at the very beginning of the workshops, when we ask people to write down the first three words that come to mind when they think about the holiday. In one workshop, ten women volunteered these typical, mixed responses: "rushed, overwhelmed, joy," "Christmas tree, happy, stressful," "rushed, children, disappointment," "fear, anticipation, excitement," "church, fun, hectic," "procrastination, joy, values," "family, Jesus, tired," "travel, excited, worried," "gifts, tree, stressful," "love, family, expectant."

One of the women in this group was surprised to find that she had written down completely opposite words. "I wrote down 'stressful' and 'happy'!" said Karen, a twenty-five-year-old artist and the mother of two young children. "And I love Christmas. Or I thought I did." Karen explained that she was excited about Christmas because it gave her a chance to make gifts for her family and get together with all of her brothers and sisters. But when she thought about why she had written down "stressful," she realized she rarely had the time to do all the things she wanted in a relaxed fashion. "I'm just starting to wrap a package when my husband walks in the door and I don't even know what I'm cooking for dinner," she said.

Karen got a better understanding of why she was always pressed for time at Christmas when we asked her to examine a list of holiday chores and check the ones that she was primarily responsible for—things like making up a gift list, shopping, sending cards, helping at church, baking, decorating, preparing for houseguests, and so forth. Karen found herself checking more than twenty items and suddenly gained a new appreciation of all the things she was trying to accomplish. (The complete list appears in the exercises at the end of this chapter.)

Like Karen, many women underestimate all the extra effort that's involved in their family celebrations. While they know full well that they are busier than usual in December, and are aware of obvious tasks like buying gifts, most of them overlook dozens of less visible chores. For example, few women stop to consider all the separate steps involved in gift giving. They often spend weeks thinking up creative gift ideas, shopping for bargains, going out of their way to specialty stores, doing original wrapping, and taking care of the mailing details. When all of their separate holiday tasks are added together, many women find that getting ready for Christmas feels like a part-time job.

One of the reasons few women realize how much extra work they do every Christmas is that they don't view most of their special chores as "work." They find an element of pleasure in almost all of them. In fact, many women look forward all year long to the holiday sewing, baking, and decorating. But what they rarely take into account is that they often have to do these things under less than ideal conditions. When they look back to the previous year, they see that they were buying gifts on lunch hours, trying to bake cookies with their children at the same time as they were cooking dinner and cleaning the house, wrapping gifts late into the night, and writing cheery notes on Christmas cards even while paying overdue bills. It's easy to see how even the most enjoyable holiday activities can become burdensome when packed into such a tight schedule.

When women see all that they're trying to do at Christmas, many of them wish for an extra two weeks. *Then* they could carry out all of their special traditions and projects and have the peace of mind to enjoy them. But few women have this luxury. They're working mothers or single parents. They have demanding careers or a houseful of children. One way or another their lives are full to begin with. And they often have to find time for Christmas by doing two things at once, staying up late, or eliminating those few unscheduled hours they count on to restore their energy.

Another aspect of their holiday role that many women fail to take into account is all the extra love and concern they pour into their families throughout the Christmas season. Women are so much more than as-sembly-line workers cranking out mince pies, wrapped gifts, and orna-ments. They also put great effort into the dozens of invisible details that make the entire season a wonderful time for the family. They plan events that will surprise and delight everyone, try to anticipate problems in the family reunion before they arise, negotiate behind the scenes with strong-willed relatives, and attempt to take into consideration each person's needs and preferences during the holiday season. And throughout it all, they buoy up all the people around them with their spirit and enthusiasm. As rewarding as all of this may be, it does require considerable thought and energy.

During the height of the holiday season, we talked with a forty-five-year old woman named Susan who gave us an indication of all the considerations that can go through a woman's mind as she prepares for her family Christmas reunion. She told us that for several days she had been cleaning the house, making the beds, shopping for groceries, and laying in a store of baked goods. And all the while she had been mentally working on solutions to the following problems: How could she tactfully persuade her husband to pay more attention to his mother-in-law? How could she entertain her fourteen-year-old niece, who was going to be the only teenager at the family reunion? How could she make life easier for her youngest sister, who had a two-year-old and a brand-new baby? How could she shield her eighty-five-year-old grandfather from the noise and chaos of so many young children? And how could she arrange the eating schedule so that her diabetic father would have small and frequent meals?

Many of the women we've talked to devote exactly this kind of emotional energy to the family Christmas. And overall, it gives them a great deal of satisfaction to put so much thought into making Christmas a wonderful time for their families. But few women give themselves full credit for all the planning, caring, and thinking involved. When women have a better sense of both the physical and the emotional demands of their holiday role, they see more clearly how their joy in the celebration can be diluted by stressful feelings: They are adding weeks of effort and devotion to an already full schedule.

For many women, these extra holiday responsibilities impose only occasional moments of stress and overtiredness. By and large, they enjoy their holiday activities, and all they may need to do to find even more enjoyment in the celebration is to look for ways to scale down their responsibilities, to become better organized, or to seek more help.

Some women, however, find that being the Christmas Magicians stirs up feelings of inadequacy as well. A woman named Chris who was raised by a hard-to-please mother told us she exhausted herself each year trying to create a perfect environment, never feeling satisfied with the results. She said, "There's this image in my head. Five little stockings hanging on the mantel. A tree decorated with gingerbread cookies and hand-sewn ornaments. But everything around me is screaming out, 'You're not measuring up! You're not measuring up!' Even my cookies don't turn out like they're supposed to."

Chris felt as if the holiday put her onstage, making all of her domestic talents—or lack of them—highly visible. The holiday seemed to test

25

her graciousness as a hostess, her diligence as a housekeeper, her artistry as a craftsman, her sensitivity as a gift giver, and her talent as a decorator. In all of these undertakings, she felt like a failure. Although some women thrive on the domestic challenge, Chris went through the season seeing everything she did through the unforgiving eyes of her mother.

Working women who try to emulate the nonstop performance of their homemaker mothers can find themselves in a similar bind. If they have fond memories of their mothers happily filling the days before Christmas with "from scratch" baking and elaborate sewing projects, they may push themselves to re-create these same good feelings for their own families—even though they work full-time outside the home. What drives them is not a fear of criticism but a desire to hand down a legacy of love to their own children. But if they fail to take into account the hectic pace of their daily lives, the result is an overcrowded schedule of projects and activities.

For other women, Christmas can stir up feelings of loneliness or anxiety. The single woman, for example, may be pained at the underlying current of family love and harmony implicit in all the Christmas specials and holiday advertising. What feels like a perfectly acceptable life the other eleven months of the year can feel like an unworkable compromise during the month of December. And women who are trying to heal from childhood wounds may find the prospect of the seasonal reunion unsettling. It's not an unmanageable gift list or a long string of holiday chores that troubles them; it's the resurrection of long-standing family conflicts.

The Christmas Machine has little tolerance for these real-life difficulties. The rest of the year, women are given a great deal of support for their various struggles, but at Christmas, all of their worries are supposed to melt away to be replaced by a surge of domestic zeal. Open up a typical December issue of a women's magazine and there's a sumptuous vision of the magical Christmas we can give our families if only we work long and hard enough. These magazines are filled with "helpful" advice on how we can transform our homes in to a winter wonderland, outdo ourselves as artists, delight everyone on our lists, dazzle the boss at the office party, and entertain with elegance and grace.

For example, one women's magazine devoted two full pages to encouraging women to fill every nook and cranny of their houses with Christmas ornaments made out of muslin. All told, the elaborate cloth creations required the combined talents of six professional artists and designers. Readers were invited to make muslin dolls, muslin Christmas stockings decorated with ribbon trellises, white-on-white ruffled coverlets and pillows, muslin baskets, and fabric trees and candles. "But don't stop there!" urged the editors. How about "lace-inset teardrop trims and soft floral triangles that repeat our stocking motifs," crowning a mantel with spectacular muslin fans and transforming muslin into a Madonna and Child?

For women who can pick and choose wisely from all of the possibilities the magazines offer, they can be a valuable resource and a welcome incentive. Holiday craft and baking projects have their definite place in the celebration—they add beauty, originality, and excitement to the holiday. But they are not essential to a good family Christmas. In fact, they can draw energy away from more important matters. What many women need to hear from the magazines is that they can give their families an equally good or even better Christmas by doing less. A friend of ours said it best: "I want to be excited by Christmas, and do a hundred projects if I feel like it. But I know that if I keep it simple, I'm not cheating myself or my family."

Ann, a working mother in her thirties, found out the hard way what her family really wanted from her at Christmas. She told us that she used to feel like a "bad mother" unless she made something from the magazines every Christmas. But two years ago she had reason to change her mind. That year she decided to make a marshmallow castle that was on the cover of a craft magazine. The directions for the castle assured her that it was a "traditional project that would add so much to a festive season" and would provide the "focal point of your holiday decorating" as well. But things didn't turn out that way.

First of all, even though the directions said that the ingredients were inexpensive, she spent over seventeen dollars at the grocery store, which was much more than she could really afford. Second, the editors claimed that the project was simple enough for a child to complete, but Ann spent ten frustrating hours putting it together. The hardest part for her was making the turrets surrounding the castle. The directions told her to paste peppermint candies to four vertical cardboard tubes with marsh-mallow crème. While the peppermints clung valiantly to the cardboard for a few hours, they oozed off during the night. When she woke up in the morning, she was greeted by a sagging castle surrounded by four half-naked toilet-paper tubes.

But the thing that really disappointed Ann was her family's reaction. She said that her husband took one look at it and told her that it was the ugliest thing he had ever seen. "He didn't even want it in the house," she said. And although the magazine told her that the "children would have hours of fun playing with the marshmallow knights and damsels that inhabit the magic castle," all *her* children wanted to do was eat them.

That experience taught her that she needed to look more carefully at her talents and interests and to be more selective about how she spent her time. "This year I'm going to spend that time with my children, instead," she said. "That's what they really want from me, anyway."

All of our interview material supports Ann's conclusion. In talking with men and children, we've found it to be invariably true that what they really want for Christmas is a house filled with love and acceptance, not a house decorated to perfection. And friends and relatives often find it refreshing to be around someone who has voluntarily taken herself out of the beautiful-house competition.

When women have an accurate picture of all that they do at Christmas and then think about what's really important to them and their families, many of them come to the conclusion that they want Christmas to be simpler. Shirley, a teacher at a Presbyterian church and the mother of four children, put it most succinctly: "I found out that I couldn't care so much about the way Christmas looked and have it feel any good."

Shirley told us that years ago she used to grab every moment of spare time to sew, bake, decorate, and write Christmas cards. "I was too busy to even question why I was doing it." But then something happened to make her examine her values. Shirley explained that her eighty-year-old mother had been living with her and was upset with herself because she didn't feel useful anymore. Her eyes were failing and she couldn't knit the kids sweaters for Christmas. She had very little money, so she couldn't buy presents for the family. "I kept telling her that she didn't have to do or buy anything," Shirley said, "that Christmas was a time to enjoy being with the family. But she wouldn't listen to me."

During that holiday season, Shirley had a revelation. "I sat down one night, absolutely exhausted from all I was doing, and took a long look at myself. There I was, trying to do all the things my mother used to do at Christmas and more. I was also busy at church. I had hardly a moment to be with my family. My own advice to my mother hit me like a sledgehammer. I suddenly realized that all that is required of us is to exist with God."

At that point, Christmas started to become a relaxed affair at Shirley's house. Instead of writing Christmas cards, she wrote one letter each Sunday of Advent to a person who had special meaning for her. She stopped trying to make the tree a thing of beauty for other people and let the children help decorate it. "Everyone laughs at me because I'm always running to a drawer on Christmas morning to get a present that I neglected to wrap. But they all have a much better time than they used to when I was a nervous wreck."

Shirley ended her story with this simple comment: "It's not that I'm lazy. If I believed it would make my family truly happy, I'd work nonstop on Christmas. It's just that I've finally realized what's important."

Shirley had strong spiritual beliefs that steered her in the direction of a simple Christmas. Most women who find ways to take the stress out of Christmas make a less dramatic change. They make one or two simple adjustments and discover that this helps them feel more in control of the celebration and gives them more energy for their traditional activities. For example, one woman who attended our workshop found that all she had to do to feel more relaxed at Christmas was to cut down on her baking. "It was the fourth pie crust that used to get to me," she said. "Now I just make one or two pies for Christmas dinner and the whole family finds that this is more than enough."

By talking with hundreds of women, we've found that there is no one holiday role that works for all women. Some enjoy the challenge of a grand celebration. Some find that a simple Christmas works best for them. And others like the freedom to vary what they do from year to year depending on their circumstances. But to make the right choice, women need a wide range of options and the freedom to define for themselves what their role is to be. In the exercises that follow, women will have a chance to examine their present holiday role and explore some possible changes. Then there are answers to specific questions women have about Christmas.

Exercises for Women

LIFE-STYLE INVENTORY

1 Many women overestimate the time they have available for holiday projects. Take the following life-style inventory to get a sense of how busy you are before you add on the responsibilities of Christmas.

> **1** Check all the following statements that are true for you:
> I'm employed full-time.
> I'm employed part-time.
> I have young children who are not yet in school or daycare.
> I have children in school or daycare.
> I'm a student.
> I'm a single parent.
> I have extended-family obligations.
> I am primarily responsible for managing the household.
> I have the following additional commitments:
> > Church
> > School
> > Volunteer work (boards, charities, committees, etc.)
> > Children's activities
> > Classes
> > Other
>
> **2** As a general rule I can count on _____hours of free time a day.
> **3** I usually spend those unscheduled hours in the following ways:
> **4** To find time to prepare for Christmas I usually take time from:

By taking this inventory, a woman named Cindy discovered that she had approximately two hours of free time a day, between nine and eleven at night. Cindy was a secretary and the mother of three children, so she often spent this time watching television or relaxing with her husband to recuperate from the routine demands on her. In order to fit in her holiday responsibilities, she had to give up this free time, try to do more than one thing at once, or stay up later than usual.

EXAMINING THE WORK OF CHRISTMAS

This exercise will help you gain a more objective view of all the holiday responsibilities you may be adding to your everyday schedule.

1 Look at the following list of typical holiday responsibilities/tasks and place a check by the ones that you were primarily responsible for last year.

* Making up a gift list
* Christmas shopping
* Making gifts
* Wrapping gifts
* Mailing gifts
* Writing cards
* Making cards
* Helping out at church
* Holiday baking
* Home decorations
* Sewing clothes
* Special holiday cleaning
* Buying stocking stuffers
* Advent preparations

* Getting the tree
* Decorating the tree
* Outside decorations
* Hosting parties
* Preparing company meals
* Helping with school activities
* Planning family gatherings
* Making Christmas dinner
* Extra grocery shopping
* Making travel arrangements
* Packing
* Preparing for houseguests
* Other

2 Add any tasks that we have overlooked.

3 Spend some time remembering how you felt last Christmas as you were doing each of the tasks that you checked. Put a star by the ones that you actually enjoyed.

4 Take a piece of paper and write down the tasks from the above list that you did not enjoy doing last year. Beside each one, write down a few words that describe the reason(s) for your dissatisfaction. Here are some common reasons:

Not enough time
Not enough money
Not enough family support
Not enough help
Don't enjoy this kind of activity
Don't value this kind of activity
My performance didn't measure up to my expectations
Wasn't creative enough

Cindy, the working mother we talked about in regard to the Lifestyle Inventory, made the following table:

Activity I didn't enjoy	Reasons
Making up gift list	Wasn't creative enough; wanted more help
Mailing gifts	Don't enjoy it; not enough time
Decorating tree	Had disagreement with my husband; tree didn't look as good as I had hoped
Cooking holiday food	Not enough time; wanted more help
Buying gifts	Not enough time or money; too many gifts; did it myself

From this exercise, Cindy learned that there were several reasons she didn't enjoy some of her traditional holiday responsibilities, but the one that came through loud and clear was that she wanted more help. Another woman took this exercise and came to a different conclusion. Her main difficulty was that she was overly critical of everything she did, so she resolved to take on fewer projects and try to be more accepting of herself.

By completing these two exercises, you now have gained a better idea of how much time you have available for holiday projects, how much you attempt to do each Christmas, and how you feel about those tasks. Later chapters will give you an opportunity to examine your values and think about how simple or elaborate you want Christmas to be. These additional considerations will help you decide whether or not you want to make any changes in your holiday role.

Questions and Answers

My family doesn't seem to notice all that I do for Christmas. Why can't they be more appreciative?

In a workshop we gave for a professional women's group, one woman told us that she thought that many of her holiday problems would vanish if she got more words of appreciation: "My fantasy is that I awake in my husband's arms, and he is kissing me and telling me how wonderful I am. How many of us hear that? 'Gee, you're wonderful. What a wonderful Christmas dinner. Thank you.' I don't hear that. I think that if we got more thank-yous, we wouldn't feel so tired."

Unfortunately, there's no way to guarantee other people's reactions to your efforts. But there are two things you can do on your own to feel better. This year, you might want to concentrate more of your energy on things that you personally enjoy doing. By finding more of your rewards in the actual process of doing things, you will find yourself less dependent on other people's responses. Second, how about trying to involve more people in the preparations? It can be frustrating to be the only person who's putting effort into the celebration. And you will probably find that the rest of your family will enjoy having a more active role to play. (The next two chapters will give you some suggestions on how to include your husband and children.)

Sometimes I wonder who's in control of my Christmas, me or my mother. I am twenty-six and I've never celebrated the holiday in my own house, even though I have a child of my own. How can I let her know that I would like to start my own traditions without hurting her feelings?

This question comes up surprisingly often. To get a better understanding of the problem, it might help if you look at the problem from both points of view. For decades, your mother has put large amounts of energy into her family Christmas, nurturing a set of family traditions that have become very important to her. To give this up and let her children start their own celebrations may feel like both a huge loss and an unwelcome reminder of her age.

You, however, are feeling the understandable need to create your own family Christmas. Having your own traditions and celebrating in your own house can be an important rite of passage. After all, this is a step that your own mother took years ago. Besides, your idea of how to celebrate Christmas may be quite different from your mother's and you may be eager for a chance to express it.

But Christmas is probably the time of year when you least want to rock the boat. Finding a workable solution will require tact and diplomacy and a keen awareness of the kind of relationship you have with your mother. If it is a frank, comfortable relationship, the best course of action may be to simply explain your desire to celebrate in your own home and then arrange another time during the holiday season (New Year's or Christmas Eve, for example) to spend time together, or invite her to come celebrate Christmas with you. Be sure to talk with her early enough in the year so that she can get used to the idea.

If you have reason to believe that your mother would not understand your wishes or would be too threatened by them, you may decide to compromise. You can continue to celebrate Christmas with her and then plan another celebration in your own home at a different time. This will allow you to start creating your own traditions and give you some of the independence you are looking for, but you will not have to openly confront your mother.

You may think of an even better way to solve this problem. Just keep in mind that your mother has sincere reasons for wanting to keep things the same and that your wish to create your own celebration is also natural and understandable.

My problem is that I don't want to give up any of my holiday activities. I enjoy them all. But I definitely get overextended. What can I do to be more relaxed?

Many women find that by starting their holiday preparations early in the year, they can do everything they want to do and still feel relaxed. For example, one woman decided to make one gift a week starting in October. By the middle of December, they were all done and she had the peace of mind to enjoy the celebration.

But many of the women we've talked to do not like to start preparing for Christmas that early. It seems unnatural to them to be working on fruitcakes and Christmas stockings in eighty-degree weather. If that's the case for you, here are two other approaches.

First, make a list of all the things that you would like to do this Christmas and arrange them in order of priority, placing the things that you absolutely have to do or most enjoy doing at the top of the list. The projects at the bottom of the list are optional, or of less importance to you.

Attack the list in order. Give yourself credit not for doing as many as possible, but for doing each project in an enjoyable fashion. Even though you may not get to the projects at the bottom of the list, you will finish most of your high-priority activities and will not feel unduly pressured.

For the second approach, you need to take a longer-range view. Each year, vow to do one or two of your favorite holiday projects. For example, this year you may decide to make a beautiful wreath for the door, as well as your own Christmas cards. The following year, you might have a neighborhood party or make some of your own gifts, without making a wreath or Christmas cards. The third year, you can do a complicated holiday baking project, making a gingerbread house with your children, but forget the other projects. This way, you will eventually get to do all that you want, but each holiday season will be more relaxed.

✳

Chapter
three

———

**MEN:
THE
CHRISTMAS
STAGEHANDS**

✳

✳

✳

✳

When we were first developing our ideas about Christmas, we gave a workshop to a group of twenty-one women at a community college in Salem, Oregon. During the first discussion period, the women talked primarily about the frantic pace of their lives at Christmas. But after lunch, they began talking about their husbands' role in the celebration. The discussion began when one woman hesitantly volunteered: "I don't know if anyone else feels this way, but my life would be a whole lot easier at Christmas if my husband helped out more. It's a one-woman show at our house. My husband used to help wrap the presents, but now he's even dropped out of that."

As soon as she had made this comment, half a dozen other women chimed in. All six of them had husbands who did very little for Christmas. In fact, after comparing notes, they were amused to find out that each husband could be counted on to do just five fairly standard holiday chores: jotting notes on Christmas cards, putting the tree in the stand, stringing the lights, mixing drinks for company, and buying gifts for his wife ("at the last minute," added one woman). The wives did the rest of the work with little or no assistance.

All of these women wanted their husbands to help out more with the holiday chores. But after exploring this idea for a while, they realized that getting help with the work load was not the most important issue. Even more than that, they wanted their husbands to be enthusiastic about Christmas and to be more emotionally involved in the family holiday activities. This last point was especially important to them, because more than anything else they wanted Christmas to bring their families closer together, while actually it often seemed to pull them apart.

These women's problems are surprisingly common. It's often the case that men are less excited about Christmas than their wives are. And women find that the season loses much of its joy when their husbands watch from the sidelines. But because they don't understand why their husbands feel cut off from the joy of Christmas in the first place, they don't know how to involve them. All they know is that the enthusiasm that comes so naturally to them is foreign to their husbands.

After two years of listening to women talk about their husbands at Christmas, we began to wonder what it would be like to hear a room full of men, not women, discussing their holiday role. Although we had always had a few men in each workshop, they were in the minority and never had a chance to explore their feelings with full male support. We decided to assemble an all-male discussion group to get a better understanding of how men really feel about Christmas.

We sent out invitations to ten thoughtful, communicative married men. In this group there were two woodworkers, an instrument maker, a construction worker, an architect, a musician, a social worker, a city planner, a truck driver, and a teacher. All but one of the men had children. Two of them had been single fathers for many years and were now remarried.

We had no idea how any of them felt about Christmas, but as we had predicted, most of them found the idea of getting together to explore their thoughts and feelings about the holiday somewhat amusing. One man exemplified the good-natured cynicism of the group when he commented: "What could men possibly have to say about Christmas? I thought it was a women's holiday."

During the first few minutes of the luncheon meeting, this light-hearted tone prevailed. But gradually the conversation grew more thoughtful. It became clear that Christmas meant more to the men than their initial comments revealed. Beneath their jokes and male camaraderie, they had strong, positive feelings about the holiday and nostalgic memories of their childhood Christmases. One man shared his early memories: "I don't recall many gifts. That's all kind of a blur. But I do remember the food. My mom would fix things she never fixed at other times. That's still really strong for me. I can remember a fruitcake that she made and little Swedish-type pastries. It was all so familiar and comforting." By thirty minutes into the meeting, the men were talking at great length about the pros and cons of telling their children the truth about Santa Claus and were revealing a deep need to feel connected with family and friends at Christmastime.

When the men got down to discussing the personal details of their family celebrations, some differences between them became apparent. One of the men, thirty-three-year-old Paul, was quite content with his family Christmas. Newly remarried, he, like his wife, viewed Christmas as an opportunity to devote more time and energy to family activities.

And to a much greater extent than the other men in the group, Paul was involved in the actual holiday preparations. "Jean doesn't get burdened with the heavy stuff," he said. "What we do, we do equally."

Twenty-eight-year-old Frank was at the other end of the spectrum. He said that he was often depressed at Christmas, and one of the reasons was that he and his wife seemed to go through the holiday on different tracks. He told the group that the previous December, his wife had stayed up sewing and baking night after night. He, on the other hand, had done his best to ignore Christmas. He had hardly given it a serious thought until December 23, and even then he had to force himself to do some last-minute shopping. "There's very little that I look forward to at Christmas," he said. "I enjoy putting up the Christmas tree. And I like to watch the kids open their gifts. But to start on a big buildup like my wife—it's just not going to happen."

Even though Frank had little enthusiasm for Christmas, he tried to hide his negative feelings from his wife. "When my wife comes running to me with her twentieth cookie recipe, I say, 'That's great.' But I'm not thinking that at all." This playacting made him feel even further removed from the festivities. He felt that Christmas was something he had to perform, and that he couldn't say what was really on his mind or do what he really wanted to do.

As soon as Frank finished talking, several of the other men made similar comments. One man remarked, "Around December first my wife starts to go on this incredible high. It's 'We gotta buy this,' 'We gotta do that,' 'We gotta fix this.' This year, she got the bright idea of refinishing the dining room floor before her parents arrived for a weekend visit. I just had to put on the armor plates and stand back. She puts out a frightening amount of energy. She gets manic and I get depressed." The man sitting to his left echoed his comments: "What you really want to do at Christmas is sit in front of the fire with your wife, or call up a few friends and have them drop by. But that's the last thing you get to do. Everything's packed into a tight schedule and it's always go, go, go." Much to his regret, Christmas seemed like an unwelcome interruption in his daily routine, a hurdle to surmount year after year.

From all of our conversations with men, we know that this group of men is a representative sample. Many men don't find the deep enjoyment they're looking for at Christmas. The holiday seems to escalate their financial worries, double their obligations, and frustrate their wishes for relaxed, intimate gatherings with family and friends. They stand back and watch their wives do most of the work and generate most of the enthusiasm, and they experience only limited enjoyment themselves. Overall, Christmas seems like an overrated family holiday that promises more than it delivers. On a scale of one to ten, few men would give Christmas more than a five.

Society gives men little encouragement to try to improve this rating. Men are expected to grumble a little about the holiday, not get too interested in the goings-on, help out when needed, and muster some enthusiasm when Christmas finally rolls around. This arm's-length attitude toward the holiday is reflected in the December issues of men's magazines. While women's magazines offer their readers a glowing vision of a wonderful Christmas, men's magazines do their best to ignore the celebration. Their only concession to the holiday is a dramatic increase in liquor ads, a photo essay on gifts for men (not what men should buy or make for other people), and the inevitable racy or cynical Christmas cartoons. The overall message to men seems to be "Drink up. The inconvenience will soon be over."

Despite this lack of encouragement, whenever we've listened to men talking at length about Christmas, they've always revealed that Christmas is very important to them. Just as much as women, they value the opportunity the holiday gives them for family togetherness, high spirits, and spiritual fulfillment, and it matters very much to them that these opportunities are realized. The men in the discussion group were no exception. As one of them summarized it, "I guess we all want Christmas to be a time of closeness and sharing. I think that is a lot of what Christ and his message are all about."

Men, as well as women, yearn for the spiritual dimension of the holiday, but the traditional male role has limited their ability to shape it. The typical husband is expected to provide financial support, help out with the errands, make a handful of suggestions, and be responsible for a few well-defined parts of the celebration. If women are the Christmas Magicians, then men are the stagehands tugging a few ropes.

Some men are fairly comfortable with the broad outlines of this role. Like their fathers before them, they expect to play a subordinate part in the celebration; and many husbands are grateful that their wives are in charge. Said one man, "I'm glad that my wife does most of the work. I could never equal her energy. I'm too laid-back." But when men explore their role in greater detail, they often find that being so uninvolved is the source of some of their dissatisfaction.

One drawback is that because they're so uninvolved in the holiday preparations, it's difficult for them to build up much interest in the celebration. When they're working hard at their outside jobs right up until the day before Christmas, they can hardly be expected to jump into the festivities with a full measure of holiday joy. In addition, their limited holiday role means that only a fraction of their talents is brought to bear on the celebration. How much pride can a man take in stringing the lights and serving the drinks? As a result, men rarely get the satisfaction of a job well done.

Second, because women often set the overall tone of the celebration, naturally relying on their own tastes, talents, and preferences, it's fairly common for their husbands' wishes to be less well represented. One of the results is that many women perpetuate their own childhood traditions to a greater degree than their husbands'. Although men may be slow to admit that their childhood Christmas traditions have much importance to them, those early experiences can have a greater impact on them than they realize. No less than their wives, men have fond memories of the specific activities and traditions of their childhood, and they derive great pleasure from reenacting them for themselves and their children. If men don't have this connection to their past, the holiday can lose a lot of its emotional appeal.

This was especially true for Ken, one of the men at the luncheon. Ken had been the single parent of three children for five years. When he had remarried, his second wife assumed full responsibility for Christmas. "And I was ready for that," he said. "I welcomed her energy." But, like most women, his wife brought with her a full complement of traditions as part of her dowry. "There was no question but that we did things her way," Ken explained. He gave an example: "When I was young, we always opened our gifts on Christmas Eve. But in my wife's family, they opened them on Christmas morning. She decided that we would open ours on Christmas morning, too. There was no compromise," he said. "Except that I compromised one hundred percent." Ken said that the first year he had opened the gifts in the morning, he felt really disoriented. "It just wasn't Christmas."

There's a final problem with men playing such a limited role in the holiday. Because men often have less decision-making power at Christmas than their wives, they sometimes feel as if they are playing a walk-on part in someone else's dramatic production. Frank, the man in the group who was often depressed at Christmas, felt this the most. "My wife calls all the shots. It's always 'Go Here.' 'Go there.' And 'You *will* go there.' I have only two choices. I can go along willingly, or I can go along reluctantly."

To one degree or another, many men we've talked to have the same feeling as Frank. It seems to them that their wives' sensibilities and social lives determine the holiday events. Women make most of the decisions about which friends and relatives to see and fill in the dates on the social calendar. Although the men have veto power, when they exercise it they are cast in a negative role.

It's clear that with women in charge, men's wishes, values, and desires are often overlooked. What would Christmas be like if the male point of view were better represented? This particular group of men wanted Christmas to be simpler and less expensive. They wanted more holiday activities that reflected their interests, more recognition of their important childhood traditions, and a stronger voice in the decision making. Many of them wanted their wives to be more relaxed and spontaneous and take on fewer holiday projects. Frank made these summary comments: "I know what my perfect Christmas would be—it would be much like it is, only I'd set aside some time to go hunting. And the rest of it would be simpler. But the most important thing is that my wife would be less wrought up, and she would ask me, 'What would *you* like to do today?' Probably it would be the same kind of thing we usually do, anyway. But it would be my choice too. And the pace would be slower."

By the end of the conversation, the men at the luncheon realized they had valid reasons for feeling left out of the festivities. They also saw for the first time that if their family celebrations were going to change for the beter, they were going to have to express their views. For many men, the key to a better Christmas is a more active role.

In recent years, this seems to be happening more and more. Men are becoming more involved in the emotional lives of their families and are becoming better acquainted with the nurturing part of themselves. This deeper involvement in family affairs promises to revitalize the celebration. As men help define Christmas, more of their values and preferences are taken into account, and as a result they become more willing to help with the details. As the work load becomes more evenly divided, busy women get a chance to relax and enjoy the celebration. Children benefit, too, because they discover they now have two enthusiastic parents with whom to share the holiday.

One couple told us how they managed to redefine their traditional roles. Tom and Cathy live in a small town where he is the director of probation services and she is a part-time social service consultant. They have two children. "In my first marriage, I felt left out of Christmas," said Tom. "I wasn't involved in the planning and I used to get pretty depressed. There were all these things I 'had to do.' I had no choice whatsoever. Marrying Cathy made all the difference. But it didn't happen automatically; we had to work on it."

One of the ways they worked at it was by listening to each other. Cathy explained: "I learned that it's important to Tom to get a lot of presents, even though it isn't to me. So now I make sure he gets lots of small, homemade gifts. And I found out that he had been depressed at Christmas for years because of money worries. So we started making all of our gifts. Tom spends long nights locked in his shop making the kids toys."

Cathy and Tom have a deep respect for each other's values, and their celebration is a blend of both of their traditions. But it wasn't always that way. As Cathy told us, "I came from a family where we have a set way of doing things. It would have been really easy for me to come to this marriage with ten billion traditions of my own. In fact, I tried to do that at first, but Tom helped me see that my ready-made Christmas was not his. Now we take the good things from my family and the good things from his family and add the things we think of ourselves."

As this story shows, warm family Christmases don't spring forth in full perfection. Husbands and wives need to talk when silence would be safer, and compromise when following one set of traditions would be easier. By respecting each other's values and feelings about the holiday and finding ways to enjoy the season together, a couple can make Christmas a time of close communion.

On the following pages, there are some simple exercises for men who want to take a closer look at their feelings about Christmas, and answers to questions that men often have about the holiday.

RATING YOUR ENJOYMENT OF LAST YEAR'S CHRISTMAS ACTIVITIES

1 Scan the list below and cross off the activities that you weren't involved in, adding those that we have overlooked.

* Decorating the house
* Decorating the tree
* Shopping for gifts
* Making gifts
* Wrapping gifts
* Entertaining
* Going to parties
* Going to Christmas performances
* Christmas activities with your children
* Christmas activities at work
* Religious activities at home
* Church activities
* Gift-opening rituals
* Charitable activities
* Family Christmas gathering
* Music
* Other

2 Beside each of the remaining activities, assign a number from 1 to 10 that shows how much you enjoyed doing it last year. A 10 shows the most pleasure. Feel free to add comments.

3 Think about what, overall, gave you the greatest pleasure last Christmas.

4 Which activities or situations gave you the least pleasure?

REMEMBERING YOUR CHILDHOOD CHRISTMAS

1 Think back to your childhood Christmas. Which traditions, activities, or occasions were particularly pleasurable for you?

2 Of these important childhood memories, which are reflected in your current celebration?

AN EXERCISE FOR MARRIED MEN—YOUR ROLE IN YOUR CURRENT CELEBRATION

1 Which of the following statements most accurately reflects your role in your celebration?

> **a** My wife determines nearly all of the holiday events.
>
> **b** My wife determines more of the holiday events than I do.
>
> **c** We share the planning fifty-fifty.
>
> **d** My influence predominates.

2 How do you feel about this arrangement?

DRAWING CONCLUSIONS

1 From everything you know about yourself and Christmas, ideally, what changes would you like to make in the coming celebration? (For the moment, don't take into consideration how realistic or unrealistic these changes may be.)

2 For married men: What do you most want your wife to know about how you feel about Christmas?

Two men who completed this exercise shared their answers with us. Steve, a thirty-seven-year-old business executive and the father of two young girls, rated his enjoyment of the previous Christmas and discovered that the activities he had enjoyed most involved his children and making gifts for other people. And the first exercise helped him realize how angry he was at all the encroaching materialism. "I feel I have to ward off the world and protect my children from the cheapening effects of commercialism."

When Steve thought about his childhood Christmas he realized that he had a wealth of happy memories. Among other things, he liked "bubble-lights on the trees," celebrating a Swedish tradition called Little Christmas on the night before Christmas, and his mother's decorating the windows with stencils.

When he thought about it, very few of his treasured traditions were being enacted in his current celebration; for example, he now opened his gifts on Christmas morning instead of Christmas Eve. The changes he wanted to make were to have more Advent rituals at home ("I like to get revved up over a long period of time"), to have more religious content in the family celebration, and to find ways of shutting out holiday commercialism. The one thing he wanted his wife to do differently was to be more sensitive to the way his family celebrated Christmas.

Arnold, a thirty-one-year-old woodworker and the father of a teenage daughter and a five-year-old son, realized that the most important thing about Christmas to him was spending relaxed time with his own family and getting together with his parents. The thing he liked least was the fact that the whole country had blown Christmas out of proportion ("It should be simple, you know") and that his own celebration seemed too tense and rushed. "I'd like to wade into Christmas Eve feeling halfway calm," he said.

His important memories of his childhood centered not so much on specific activities but on the whole aura of relaxed calm that his family had cultivated at Christmas. "There was no pressure. There was no worrying about money. It was simple and under control."

Arnold was often depressed by the frantic pace of Christmas, and wanted very much to scale things down and for his wife to be less busy. He wanted her to take on only projects that she could do comfortably. And he wished that he had more time off from work to take part in the Christmas activities in a leisurely fashion.

In the remaining chapters of this book, men will have a chance to explore other aspects of Christmas and to clarify any changes they might want to make in the celebration.

Questions and **A**nswers

I don't think I've been genuinely happy at Christmas since I was a child. What's wrong?

Some time during the transition from childhood to full adulthood, Christmas begins to change for people. The magic and surprise and beauty of Christmas are tempered by all the careful thought and work and expense that they put into the happiness of others. For many people this transition is accelerated by the birth of their own children. At that point they step over the line separating the Christmas recipients from the Christmas providers.

But even given this inevitable change in feelings, you can still find a deeper and more mature satisfaction in the holiday. The first thing you need to do is to accept the fact that, as an adult, you will rarely experience Christmas in the same way you did as a child. When you let go of that universal desire to be young at Christmas, you will make room for the new kind of pleasure you can find as an adult.

Also, as we said in the body of this chapter, you will probably find that your enjoyment of Christmas is increased if you carry over some traditions from your childhood into your current celebration. You won't feel exactly the same way about them as you did when you were young, but your Christmas will be enriched by the memories of all those that have gone before.

Finally, reading this chapter and doing the exercises have probably given you some important information about other ways to increase your enjoyment of Christmas. We have talked with men who have gone from being depressed at Christmas to finding it one of the most enjoyable parts of the year. They did this by actively seeking a new role that matches their personalities and beliefs.

How can I enjoy Christmas when I'm so busy at work that I hardly have time to turn around?

If you have the luxury, take a few days off from work at Christmas. One man that we talked to had had to take a week off one Christmas because his office shut down to do some remodeling. He enjoyed Christmas so much more that year that he has taken a vacation at the end of December ever since.

If taking time off at Christmas isn't practical, even a few unscheduled hours of leisure time can restore your spirits and replenish your energy for the things you want to do for the holiday. You might want to cancel your usual meetings or delay activities you generally enjoy—bridge games, bowling, night classes—until January.

Finally, you may want to eliminate some of your usual holiday activities. Many men find that they would rather give up a tradition than do it in a rushed, frantic way. By scaling down your obligations, you will have more time and peace of mind to enjoy the ones that remain. (Later chapters will help you simplify your celebration.)

My wife and I often fight over money at Christmas. What should we do?

Both men and women are placed in awkward positions at Christmas. Men are given the message that their success as husbands and fathers depends on how much money they make available for the family Christmas. But on the other hand, they are typically excluded from many of the actual decisions about how that money is spent. In most cases, their wives are the ones who choose the gifts and write the checks. Men are often left out of this process until they are presented with the final bill. Understandably, many men are upset by the fact that their primary function is to provide the funds and that they have so little control over how they're spent.

Women may not only be contributing to the family income, but also carrying most of the responsibility for deciding how the money should be spent. They are the ones who have to make sure that Aunt Hattie has her customary gift, that the dinner lives up to everyone's expectations (her husband's included), and that the children are suitably outfitted for the Holiday Review at Grandma's. And women are often the only ones in their families who fully realize how much these things cost. When their husbands open the bills, the men are often unaware of all the careful planning and bargain hunting that went into keeping the totals as low as they are. All they see is that Christmas costs way too much.

Understanding this double bind is the first step in resolving the problem. Even when a couple chooses to keep the traditional financial arrangement, they profit from consulting each other more frequently during the holiday season so that both of them are aware of the total monetary picture.

But poor communication is not the only source of financial tension at Christmas. More and more people are coming to the conclusion that they are simply spending too much money. No matter who's making the decisions and who's making the money, spending can get out of hand. In every chapter of this book you will find specific suggestions for trimming your expenses.

In addition to adjusting the total amount of money they are spending, many people see the need for more conscious financial planning at Christmas. They want to know ahead of time how much money they have available and ensure that that money is spent on things they value. A simple holiday budget plan that may help can be found in the Appendix.

Every Christmas I feel a little down. How can I keep from being so depressed?

Like you, a lot of people go through the holiday season feeling sad and unhappy just when they want to feel their best. There may be any number of reasons for your unhappiness. You may have family problems. You may be worried about money. You may have health problems or job concerns. Or you may be lonely. Unfortunately, problems don't disappear at Christmas, and many people find that they are intensified. We want so much to be lighthearted and gay that the bad moods we can cope with at other times of the year seem unmanageable during the holiday season.

Some people find that their depression feeds on itself. In the beginning, they are unhappy for a specific reason. Then they are upset at themselves for being unhappy at Christmas. And they may also resent the real or imagined pressure from those around them to be in a better mood. All of this can turn a mild case of the blues into a black mood.

There are several things you can do to raise your spirits. First, stop putting unreasonable pressure on yourself to be happy at Christmas. Despite appearances, most people are no more or less happy at Christmas than at any other time of the year. And when you have legitimate reasons for being unhappy, acknowledge them.

Second, you may find that your bad mood improves when you're in the company of special friends and favorite relatives—especially those who accept your full range of feelings and don't put pressure on you to be other than you are. So seek out people who make you feel better, and avoid people who contribute to your depression.

Third, make an effort to be more physically active. Physical activity is one of the best antidotes to depression. Research indicates that exercise stimulates the production of endorphins, mood-elevating chemicals produced by the body. Take a walk, go to the gym, get out in the country, or take on a project that calls for physical activity.

Fourth, many people recover their equilibrium when they set one or two specific, manageable goals every day—even if they are as simple as cleaning out a closet or writing a letter. The satisfaction they get from completing these tasks adds to their sense of well-being and self respect.

How can I get my wife to slow down and enjoy Christmas? She's running nonstop from Thanksgiving to New Year's.

If the two of you sit down early in November and talk about what's most important to you at Christmas, it will be easier to set some priorities. Clearly, one of your goals is to have more relaxed time together with your wife. When she understands how important her company and peace of mind are to you, she will have more incentive to trim the "To Do" list. One way to take the weight off her shoulders is to develop a core list of all those activities you both agree are essential to the enjoyment of the season, and then divide up the necessary tasks. Your increased involvement will be greatly appreciated, and the two of you will have more time to relax and enjoy the beauty of Christmas as a result.

※

*Chapter
four*

———

**THE
FOUR THINGS
CHILDREN
REALLY WANT
FOR
CHRISTMAS**

※

※

※

※

Deborah, a twenty-nine-year-old homemaker, lives with her husband and her son Alex in a trailer in a remote rural area. Deborah told us that her most enjoyable Christmas had been the year before, when Alex was three. At first as we listened to her describe that particular holiday, it seemed more like a disaster than a memorable celebration. She and her husband had had very little money to spend on gifts and had had to scrimp and save just to buy candles and baking supplies. Then Deborah had spent the entire week before Christmas in bed with the flu which had forced them to cancel all their visits with family and friends. All the same, it had been a wonderful Christmas because of Alex. "He was the perfect age to be excited by Christmas," she said. "It took so little to please him. His favorite gift of all was a one-dollar race car he found in his stocking. He played with it all morning." She said that for the first time since she was a child, she had felt real joy at Christmas.

When the two of us became parents, we, too, were more excited about the holiday than we had been in years. We found that we looked forward to Christmas morning with the same eagerness that we had felt twenty-five years earlier, only this time we were excited about the gifts our children would unwrap, not about anything we would receive. And our children gave us a wonderful excuse to bring out the forgotten artifacts of our childhood—the Advent calendars, Christmas books, and angel chimes. Being the parents of young children gave us back some of the lost magic of Christmas.

The parents who come to our workshops have this same desire for a rich, family-centered celebration, and they're eager for suggestions on how to give their children a wonderful Christmas. But some of them bring other concerns as well, because in addition to the joy children bring to Christmas, they can also bring added complications. One concern voiced by most parents is that of shielding their children from the excesses of holiday commercialism. While adults can mute the TV when the ads get annoying, children are defenseless against the onslaught of ads. As early as the age of four or five, they can lose the ability to be delighted by the sights and sounds of Christmas, only to gain a two-month-long obsession with brand-name toys. Suddenly, all they seem to care about is how many presents they will be getting and how many days are left until they unwrap them.

We've run across this problem in every workshop we've ever given, but one woman's story stands out in our memory. Shelley, the mother of a nine-year old-boy named John, came to one of our seminars bringing her son's letter to Santa. When she held up the letter, we saw two pages filled with his schoolboy's scrawl. All told, he had requested over sixty gifts, most of them brand-name toys.

Shelley was clearly troubled by John's letter. A devout Christian, she was appalled that he was so locked into the "gimme" side of the celebration. She blamed his mania for gifts on his friends, television commercials, and store displays. Everything seemed to conspire to make him greedy, and she felt defeated in her efforts to teach him better values.

Like Shelley, many parents find it a challenge to create a simple, value-centered Christmas in the midst of all the commercial pressure. But the task is made much easier when parents keep in mind the four things that children really want for Christmas. While children may be quick to tell their parents that what they want is designer clothes, the latest electronic gear, and brand-name toys, underneath these predictable requests is an unspoken plea for four, more basic requirements:

1 A relaxed and loving time with the family.
2 Realistic expectations about gifts.
3 An evenly paced holiday season.
4 Reliable family traditions.

These basic needs play the determining role in whether or not children have a good family Christmas. Let's explore them one by one. The first requirement on this list—a relaxed and loving time with the family—probably comes as no surprise to you. Even more than gifts, children want love at Christmas. Dr. Patricia Love, director of the Austin Family Institute, underscores this point: "What children really want at Christmas—just like at any time of the year but more so during the holiday season—is time with their parents. A parent's relaxed, freely

Dear Santa Please Bring me

1. Danvan
2. Race and chace
3. Roket
4. Spiderman set
5. Crayons
6. Cow Boy suit and hat and Boots, gun
7. Fishing pole
8. Clothes - size - 7 shirt   22. Big elgo
9. Big Deteour Racetrack   23. foot Ball
10. Dead Stop game   24. ha noman
11. match Box Garage   25. Spiderman
12. Bigtrack   26. Ravon Shawn
13. micky. mouse clock   record
14. einstine game   27. major merega
15. the amaricon Dream game   28. crash up darby
16. Teddy Bear   29. star tek micro
17. Lunch Box   30. Pro Thunder
18. Coot   Bike
19. Radio   31. Alien monster
20. Socer Ball
21. mouse trap game

52

33. Saturday Night Fever Record
34. Coloring Book
35. Electric Battleship
36. Super tuber
37. Intercept
38. AM Speedsteer
39. Be Be gun
40. I tokin Space
41. Maxmachine Nighthawk
43. Shasam Underoos
44. Stratego
45. Glow in the dark Shrinkidinks
46. Increadable Hulk instant muscles
47. Energise Spiberman set
48. Downfall
49. Slapsie
50. Layan egg game
51. knockout game
52. Bowling Ball
53. Skidoo

53. Superstar 3000
54. Sit and spin
55. Suckerman
56. ROM
57. walk and Talking pack RACE
58. Hit and misste
59. Ranger TV
60. Hot weeds
61. Torture chamber
62. Drum set
63. Attack!

given attention conveys a simple but profound message: "You are a priority in my life."

Ironically, many parents find it more difficult to spend relaxed time with their children in December than at other times of the year. Shelley, the mother of the boy with the foot-long gift list, was a prime example. Despite her love for her son, she was rarely available to him in those hectic weeks before Christmas. She worked full-time as a seamstress in a swimsuit factory, and in December her evenings were crowded with holiday chores. Her husband was also busier than usual because he was a salesman in a sporting goods store, and the store made as much as third of its annual sales between Thanksgiving and Christmas. Because of his many hours of overtime, he, too, had little time to spend with his son. During our workshop Shelley came to the realization that one of the reasons her son spent so much time daydreaming about gifts was that he was often left to his own devices during the evenings, and that usually meant sitting in front of the TV.

As was true for Shelley and her husband, many parents find that their lives become crowded with holiday obligations during the month of December. Even though they shower their children with gifts and affection on Christmas Day, a feeling of emptiness remains. Children want love in a steady, constant way.

Some parents deprive their children of their relaxed attention at Christmas for the opposite reason: They are worn out from their efforts to make the month of December a flurry of family events. They take their children to the store displays, the *Nutcracker* ballet, breakfast with the Cinnamon Bear, Santa's helicopter's arrival at the mall, and the seasonal tour of decorated houses. To this crowded roster, some well-intentioned parents add a trip to a nursing home, a visit to the Salvation Army to deliver canned goods, and a full complement of church-sponsored activities. No wonder the parents' nerves are a little frayed as they lace their children into their red-and-green velvet matching outfits to make the annual journey to Grandma's.

To create just the right balance between family activities, community events, and just plain "hanging-out" time, parents need to pay close attention to their own needs and to the needs of their individual children. Anna, the single mother of a three-year-old boy named Jeffrey, recounted the time when she was made aware of just how hard she was pushing to give her family The Perfect Christmas. One Saturday just before Christmas she was busily cleaning the house to get ready for her parents' annual visit. She spent all day mopping and waxing the floors, scrubbing the bathroom, washing the linens, making the beds, washing the windows, and baking bread. She wanted the house to glow when her parents walked in the door. Her son, Jeffrey, of course, had no interest in her ultimate goal; he just wanted attention.

After sending Jeffrey to his room to cool off from his second full-blown tantrum, Anna took a deep breath and examined her priorities. What was more important, she asked herself, rushing to make a dessert or spending some time with Jeff. She decided to forgo the dessert. She went into Jeffrey's room and asked if he wanted to bundle up and go for a walk with her. Suddenly, he was all smiles. Anna and Jeffrey spent an hour poking around the woods next to the house and came home with an armload of branches and berries to make a centerpiece for the dining room table. The dessert never did get made, but mother and son were both in good spirits when the grandparents' car pulled into the driveway.

In addition to this moment-by-moment appraisal of daily events, many parents find that it helps to do some long-range planning. We talked with a couple from Colorado who found the only way they could spend relaxed time with their children was to turn down all social invitations after mid-December. To make sure this would happen, they got out the calendar the day after Thanksgiving and drew a red-and-green box around the days from December 15 to January 1. They vowed that nothing was going to intrude on this space. Another woman told us that Christmas had gotten so hectic she had to tell her relatives that her family wouldn't be traveling for Christmas—even though she risked offending them. Both of these families had decided that family time was top-priority, and they were well rewarded by their children's deep enjoyment of Christmas.

The second unspoken plea children make each Christmas is to have realistic expectations about gifts. No child wants those long weeks of anticipation to end in disappointment. Unfortunately, parents are not the only ones shaping their children's expectations. Watching television on a typical Saturday morning in December, a child may see from fifty to sixty toy commercials using the most sophisticated techniques Madison Avenue has at its disposal—stunning graphics, unforgettable jingles, appealing child actors, and dramatic camera shots. As any parent knows, those ads can be amazingly effective. One father told us about the time his six-year-old son was watching a commercial for a popular board game. When it was over, his son turned to him and said, "I want that game for Christmas." The father explained there was nothing unusual about his son's asking for a toy that had just been advertising—he did that all the time. But this case was different. "We had that game already," said the father, "and my son was bored to tears with it. The commercial sold him on something we already owned."

Children are one of the prime targets of the Christmas Machine because toys are the most dependable part of the holiday trade. No matter how little money people have, they will always find a way to buy toys for their children. And advertisers learned long ago that it is more effective to target their toy commercials at children than at the parents who ultimately do the buying. The following comments are from a July 19, 1965, article in an advertising trade journal entitled *Advertising Age*. "When you sell a woman on a product and she goes into the store and finds your brand isn't in stock, she'll probably forget it. But when you sell a kid on your product, if he can't get it, he will throw himself on the floor, stamp his feet, and cry. You can't get a reaction like that from an adult."

What can parents do about all the commercial pressure? Children need the security of knowing that the family, not Madison Avenue, is in control. For this to be the case, parents may have to counter some of the messages their children have absorbed from the media or from talking to other children. A good way for them to do this is to be explicit about what kind of gifts their children will be receiving. As an example, a parent might say to a seven-year-old child, "This year, you will be getting two presents from me, one big one—like the bike I gave you last year—and one smaller one, like a board game or video game." This helps keep their expectations in line with reality.

If a child asks for a gift that is not in keeping with the family budget, it's important that parents convey that information. They need to show that they understand the desire for the present, but also that they have financial limits. A parent might say to a teenage child, "I agree that new skis and boots would be fun, but money is tight right now. You'll have to think of something that costs less." If a child asks for a gift that

*The
four things
children
really want
for
Christmas*
✳

is inappropriate for some other reason, a wise mother or father will explain why. "I know you would really like a puppy, Suzanne, but no one is home during the day to take care of it. Can you think of a pet that would do well alone?"

Some of the parents who come to our workshops express a desire to give their children fewer gifts than they have in the past. A mother of two teenage boys told us why she had decided to scale back her gift giving. In the past, she had given her boys big-ticket items like stereos and ski equipment. "I wanted them to know they were the most important people in the world to me," she told us. "But the only message they got was 'Mother spent a lot of money.' I'm not going to do that anymore." We advised her to tell her boys as soon as possible about her decision to cut back and to explain her reasons. Then we suggested she give them something else to look forward to, such as a trip or favorite family activity. This way they could focus on what they would be getting, not on what they would not.

Parents with young children can help their sons and daughters keep their expectations in line with reality by arming them with more defenses against the ads. Studies have shown that many children five years and younger cannot distinguish between commercials and regular programming. Even older children can be duped when a cartoon show is based on characters that have been exploited into a whole line of products, because, in effect, the show itself has become a feature length ad. Watching the *Teenage Mutant Ninja Turtles* for half an hour is the same thing as watching a thirty-minute ad for the scores of its spin-off products. According to Peggy Charron, longtime TV reformer, toy manufacturers turned more than seventy such toys into TV series during the 1980s, "creating a toy promotion bonanza for the advertiser."

An effective way to protect young children from this commercialism is to watch an hour of children's television with them. Have the youngest ones say, "Commercial!" each time a new one comes on the screen. Then talk about each ad on a level that is appropriate for the age of the child. What is being advertised? How are the products made to seem especially inviting? We've talked with children as young as four years old who could tell us that the purpose of advertising is to sell things, and that the toys are rarely as enticing as the ads make them appear. Older children can be challenged to count the number of commercials in an hour or to time the length of typical ads. The more children are able to analyze the commercials, the less vulnerable they will be to the messages.

The third unspoken request children have at Christmas is to have an evenly paced holiday season. Ideally, they would like to participate in family activities spaced throughout a one- or two-week period, not spend months waiting for a celebration that is over in a few hours of frenzied gift unwrapping. In essence, they are making a plea for the kind of holiday season that was celebrated before the advent of the Christmas Machine when there was a shorter buildup to Christmas and a longer period of family games and festivities once the holiday officially arrived.

This wish for a more natural holiday season will not happen without parental intervention. As we mentioned in earlier chapters, retailers jump the gun on Christmas because of their desire to extend the holiday shopping season as long as possible. Unfortunately, as any parent knows, as soon as a child sees the first cardboard Santa in a grocery store, the long countdown to Christmas begins. Today's kids may have a ninety-day buildup to Christmas in which they have little to do but watch Christmas specials on TV and count off the days on the calendar.

When Christmas finally arrives, it's over before it begins. Commercial interests pack up their decorations, rented Santas, and Christmas carols on December 26 because the selling season is over. If families follow the commercial calendar, they, too, have nothing to offer children after Christmas Day. When the gifts are unwrapped, Christmas is over and the children are left dazed and bewildered.

One mother told us that she found her daughter crying in the closet on Christmas Day—just after she had opened all the gifts she had asked for. When the worried mother asked her daughter what was wrong, the girl answered, "If I had known this was all there was to Christmas, I wouldn't have waited so long."

Judith, a seven-year-old girl from Los Angeles, gave us another glimpse of the child's view of Christmas. "I have to wait two billion years for Christmas," she told us. "When it comes, it only lasts a second. Then the whole world is plain again." Being a resourceful child, Judith decided to take matters into her own hands. She confided to us that she had written a letter to Santa, asking him "to take an early run to my house. About November 10." She told her parents that Santa had agreed. "I went a little too far with that one," she confessed.

It's easier than most parents think to give their children a more natural holiday season. All they have to do is hold off on their important family traditions until a few weeks before Christmas, and then reserve a few favorite ones to add joy and meaning to the remaining days of Christmas vacation. Here's how one family does it. On December 15, they celebrate the beginning of Christmas by getting out their Christmas records. On the following weekend, they drive to the country to scavenge materials to make a wreath for the front door. On December 20, they put up their tree. The day after Christmas they invite the grandparents over for brunch. And on January 1, they wind down the celebration with a traditional potluck dinner for their friends and their children.

The children are so secure in this order of things that they have no difficulty with the premature holiday displays. In fact, the father told us that he was in the grocery store one day in early November with his daughters, and the girls saw the manager hanging some plastic holly over the cash registers. In a loud voice, the youngest girl piped up: "What's he doing that for? Doesn't he know that Christmas is a long way away? We haven't even gotten out the music, yet."

There's a final need children have at Christmas, and that's to have a celebration enriched with family traditions. Many parents underesti- mate how important traditions are to their children and how many valuable purposes they serve. First of all, traditions give children some- thing to look forward to year after year, which is of great significance to them. One mother told us that for several years she and her boys had made a gingerbread house each Christmas. One year she suggested that they make a permanent one instead, but her boys would have no part of it. To them, it just wasn't Christmas if they couldn't make a ginger- bread house every year.

Second, traditions enrich each holiday with the memory of all the Christmases that have gone before. Each year that a mother pulls the same recipe out of the card file and invites the children to help her with the baking, each year the same relatives or family friends are invited for New Year's brunch, each year the family gathers in front of the piano and sings the same songs from the family collection of Christmas carols, the children recall the many times they have enacted these rituals before. The experience becomes a rich mixture of overtones.

Finally, traditions give children great comfort. When many of their routines are disrupted by the holiday season—school is out, their parents

59

may be unusually busy, and everyday schedules fall by the wayside—children like to cling to well-defined rituals which give them a welcome sense of order and the security of knowing exactly how the season will unfold.

Traditions become especially important when there is a major transition in the family, whether through a move, a divorce, a death in the family, or a remarriage. With a major change to adapt to, familiar activities are especially important. A recently widowed friend of ours with a four-year old boy found this to be true. Before she and her son had their first Christmas alone together, she asked her son what he remembered most about the previous Christmas. "That Santa on a string" was his cryptic reply. She was puzzled for a moment until she realized he was referring to a simple, two-dimensional Santa Claus ornament that had hung at his eye level on the tree the year before. "That ornament meant nothing to me," she said. "I could easily have tucked it away in favor of something grander. I'm glad I bothered to ask." Later, she discovered that her son also wanted the Advent calendar placed in the exact same spot it had been placed the year before. When she started to pin the calendar up on a different wall, the boy pointed to the old spot and said, "No, Mommy. You goofed. It always goes over there." She quickly hung the calendar in its familiar place. In these simple ways, she was able to satisfy her son's heightened need for routine.

Although traditions are a key ingredient of the holiday season, parents don't have to run to the library and check out books on holiday customs or struggle to invent elaborate new rituals. As the above story illustrates, children perceive anything they can count on year after year as a tradition, and most families have more of these hidden rituals than they realize. The holiday food they make every year, the customary invitations extended to family and friends, the familiar faces at the Christmas dinner table, the same favorite decorations, the records and books that come out each December, the way the Christmas cards are displayed—all of these things become landmarks in a child's celebration. All parents need to do is talk with their children to find out which holiday rituals are most important to them, and make an effort to do them each year.

Once parents understand the four things children really want for Christmas—relaxed time with their families, realistic expectations about gifts, an evenly paced holiday season, and reliable family traditions, they can create a joyful and enduring celebration. No matter how many products the children see advertised on TV, and no matter how many gifts their friends may receive, their parents will be giving them the most lasting gift of all—a joyful, family-centered Christmas.

To adapt these ideas to your unique situation, complete the following exercises. Then scan through the list of common questions parents have about Christmas. (Gift ideas for children appear in the Appendix in the back of the book.)

Exercise

HELPING CHILDREN ENJOY CHRISTMAS
1 Of all the needs of children at Christmas, enjoyable time with their families is most important. Think back to last December. *Excluding* Christmas Eve and Christmas Day, did you spend (underline the correct word) more, about the same, or less, happy, relaxed time with your children in December, compared to other months?
2 If your answer to the above question was "less," look through the following list and check the suggestions on how to spend more time with your children that seem most feasible for you.

* Taking extra time off from work
* Simplifying our holiday preparations
* Entertaining less
* Attending fewer parties that are just for adults
* Being more relaxed about how the house looks
* Cutting back on outside commitments
* Making fewer gifts
* Watching less television
* Traveling less
* Seeing fewer friends and relatives
* Other

3 Which holiday traditions do your children seem to enjoy most? (If you are uncertain, take some time in the next few days to talk with them.)

4 What holiday traditions or family activities do your children have to look forward to after December 25? (If you have none or very few, see pages 72–73 for some suggestions.)

5 Check the statement that most accurately completes this thought: Gift giving plays the following role in our family celebration:

> ✳ It is by far the most important tradition.
> ✳ It is one of several important traditions.
> ✳ It is of moderate importance.
> ✳ It is of relatively minor importance.

6 On a sheet of paper, write each of your children's names and jot down a few sentences that describe each child's attitude toward Christmas presents last year. (If one or more of your children seemed overly concerned with gifts, you may wish to review this chapter.)

Questions and Answers

I'm recently divorced. How can my children and I have a good Christmas?

Single parents have a lot to contend with at Christmas. Their own feelings of failure and loss are intensified by a celebration that stirs up powerful memories and glorifies the advantages of the traditional family. They must wrestle with these private doubts and sorrows at the same time as they are reassuring their children (who are also coping with the loss of a parent) that all the joy and excitement of Christmas will be theirs. And they must do all of the work involved in providing a good family Christmas by themselves. It's no wonder that many single parents ask whether a good Christmas is possible.

Without denying how difficult Christmas for a single parent can be, we assure you that a good Christmas is within your reach. We've met many single-parent families that find Christmas one of the best times of the year. It may help you to keep in mind that over 20 percent of all American families are headed by single parents. It is our *stereotyped image* of the family at Christmas that is out of sync, not the single-parent family itself. It may also help you to remember that married people are not exempt from problems at Christmas, either.

But beyond these realizations, here are some additional suggestions for creating a sense of wholeness at Christmas. First, accept the fact that yours is not a traditional family at Christmas. This acceptance is the necessary first step. The desire to get together again with your ex-spouse can be overwhelming, but the single parents and family counselors we've talked to say it's usually a mistake. Pretending you're a united family again is usually depressing for the adults and confusing for children (although they may ardently desire it), and it delays your progress in finding a new family identity. You need to believe—and demonstrate—that your new family is capable of growing and loving and having fun at Christmas just the way it is.

Second, encourage your children to spend enjoyable time with both parents during the holidays, if possible. Your attitude here is crucial. If either you or your spouse acts left out and full of self-pity, the children may feel guilty. But if you cooperate in making the arrangements and encourage your children to participate enthusiastically in the holiday activities of both parties, Christmas can be a joyful time for them. Some of the children we've talked to even consider themselves lucky because they have two celebrations.

Most single parents tell us how important it is to get these arrangements with ex-spouses made in advance. If visiting arrangements can become traditions, the children gain a sense of security, you are relieved of debilitating negotiations with your ex-spouse, and a definite yearly rhythm is established for the holidays.

Third, plan your own Christmas activities ahead of time. Don't drift through the holidays waiting for something wonderful to happen to you, and don't overload your schedule with Christmas obligations that crowd out the activities you value. Ask yourself what you really need this Christmas to balance the rest of your life. If you need to get away, then consider how you might finance a trip. If you need more social interaction, send out invitations to a party. If you need a more realistic perspective on your own problems, arrange to get involved with those less fortunate. If you need time with your own children, decline other invitations—even if it means breaking with old traditions.

But one note of caution: Don't expect all your planning to make

Christmas perfect. Even the most carefully thought-out celebration is subject to the same ebb and flow as everyday living. One woman told us, "I'm trying to broaden my understanding of what a celebration is. Rather than trying to keep all the holes corked and the windows shut and arranging for the hermetic encirclement of the house, I'm trying to allow all of us more freedom."

Fourth, initiate new traditions. One of the most striking things about Christmas is its power to pull you into the past. Something as innocuous as a certain kind of wrapping paper can trigger memories that flood you with feelings you thought you had forgotten. For most people, these memories are pleasant; but for a newly divorced person, they can be a burden. For example, one minister came up to us during a break in a workshop and admitted that talking about Christmas was painful for him. "My wife left me ten months ago and took the kids. Every time you use the words 'family' and 'Christmas' together, I feel like crying. It's all the memories."

Most single parents find that their battle with the Ghost of Christmas Past is easier when they are protected by a shield of new traditions. Old memories don't sting as much when everyone is involved in new activities that signal a new beginning for the family.

Take a look at your Christmas traditions with fresh eyes. Do you really enjoy all the rituals that have become second nature to you at Christmas, or have they become habits? Do they carry meaning for you? Do they suit your new circumstances? One single mother answered no when she asked herself about the traditional Christmas Eve dinner she used to prepare for eight people. It just didn't make sense for her new family of three. So she and her two daughters have begun a new tradition—takeout pizza on Christmas Eve.

Fifth, beware of overdoing the presents to your children. It's natural for many single parents to feel some guilt about their children during and after a divorce. And it's a temptation to try to compensate with Christmas presents. But our conversations with child psychiatrists, single parents, and children themselves show that what children really need from Christmas in times of family stress is the reassurance that they are loved, and the security of knowing that they can grow and learn and be happy in their family just like a child in any other family.

With time, most single parents discover for themselves that overloading their children with presents isn't necessary or even desirable. As one man told us, "I used to feel guilty about being a single father at Christmas. I knew I couldn't provide what a mother could, so I spent a zillion dollars on Christmas presents. Now I know I didn't have to do that. Jesse was getting enough just by my loving him."

What are some ways my young children and I can have a good time together this holiday season?

One of the easiest and most rewarding things you can do is to take a look at your existing holiday activities and see if your children have an active role to play in them. All too often at Christmas, children are the passive recipients of their parents' labors. Then, make sure that you are in a relaxed, accepting frame of mind as you take part in seasonal activities. A common tendency is for the look of the finished product to become more important than the act of creating it. One mother told us that she had a wonderful time baking cookies with her children and doing craft projects at every time of year except Christmas. Then, suddenly, she became preoccupied with making *beautiful* cookies and *beautiful* ornaments, so her children were just in the way.

One mother had a refreshingly different point of view: "I let the kids decorate the cookies with me last year with the frosting that comes in tubes. And you'd better believe those cookies had FROSTING. They looked terrible. They tasted terrible. But they were great."

To help eliminate any tension in your baking sessions, you might want to save your complicated recipes for times when the kids aren't around. You could use store-bought refrigerator cookie dough and let the kids decorate the slices with red and green sprinkles or icing from tubes. Or, if you want to make your goodies from scratch, here are two recipes that are simple enough for preschoolers.

✳ ————————————————————————————

APRICOT NUT BALLS

12 TO 18 BALLS

1 *cup chopped apricots (1 6-ounce package)*
½ *cup dried coconut*
½ *cup graham cracker crumbs (3 to 4 double crackers)*
1 *to 2 tablespoons sweetened condensed milk (not evaporated)*
½ *cup chopped nuts (you can buy them chopped)*

Put everything but the nuts into a bowl. Mix with a spoon. Shape into balls, logs, or cookies. Roll in the chopped nuts. Refrigerate until served.

Following is a simple no-bake fruitcake that uses dried fruit in place of candied fruit.

NO-BAKE FRUITCAKE

1 LOAF

❋

2 cups graham cracker crumbs (14 double crackers)
1 cup chopped nuts (you can buy them chopped)
1¼ cups chopped, mixed dried fruit (1 6-ounce package; also available chopped)
1 14-ounce can sweetened condensed milk (not evaporated)

Put all the dry ingredients into a bowl. Mix with your hands or a spoon. Add the condensed milk and stir. Line a bread pan with plastic wrap or waxed paper. Press the dough into the pan. Cover with paper and press again. Refrigerate. Then slice and serve.

Making salt-dough ornaments is another wonderful holiday activity for children, because they can mold and shape the clay to their heart's content and then, when it's dry, have the additional fun of painting it. Here's a good recipe. The ingredients are inexpensive and you probably have everything you need without making a special trip to the store.

BAKER'S CLAY

❋

2 cups white flour
1 cup salt
1 cup water (warm water feels good to the hands)
2 tablespoons oil

Combine all the ingredients. Knead for 10 minutes or until smooth. (If the dough is too crumbly, add water. If it's too moist, add flour.) Roll and cut with cookie cutters or shape into snow people, gingerbread men, or whatever. Bake in a 325°F oven until dried, but not browned (about 15 minutes per ¼ inch).

When cool, paint with watercolors, acrylic paint, or felt pens. Spray with plastic for a more durable, shinier surface.

Note: If you want to hang these ornaments on the tree, insert a bent paper clip through the top before baking them.

Sprinkled throughout the rest of this chapter and in the others as well, you will find more easy projects and activities to do with your children. But the crucial element in all of them is a relaxed and accepting parent.

I feel that our Christmas celebration lacks meaningful traditions. How can we find good ones to add?

Whether yours is a young family just beginning to create its own holiday traditions or a more established family that wants to add some new ones, the first place we suggest you look is in your own childhood memories. Try to recall a few significant Christmases and remember which events or activities gave you the most pleasure. How many of those traditions are included in your current celebration? If you are married, have your spouse do the same thing. You and your children will get added pleasure from knowing that your traditions have a history.

Another place you might want to look for traditions is in your parents' or grandparents' childhood Christmases. Sit down with them and have them tell you about their early holiday memories. The joy of reaching into the past and rescuing a forgotten tradition can illuminate the lives of every generation in your family.

Beyond that, you might wish to explore your ethnic heritage. Many of our most vital folk traditions are being slowly extinguished in favor of more homogeneous, commercialized activities. There are dozens of books in your public library to aid you in your research. Or, once again, call on your oldest surviving family members.

Remember that your holiday traditions can be quite simple. One family we know has made a tradition out of opening their Christmas cards. Each day, the unopened cards are placed in the center of the Advent wreath. After dinner, all three children choose cards to open. They look carefully at the illustrations, pass them around the table, and then listen while their parents read the messages inside and tell them a little about the people who sent them. This is one of the favorite traditions of all the family members, and it costs nothing, involves no preparation time, and teaches the children a little about the special people in their lives.

The toy commercials on television really bother me. What else can I do to protect my children from them?

One thing you can do is become more knowledgeable about what effect television advertising and television in general have on your children. Here's a good book for more information: *TV Smart Book for Kids* by Peggy Charron and Carol Hulsizer (New York: E.P. Dutton, 1986).

Second, you can limit your children's television hours. The average child spends four hours a day watching TV, more time than they spend studying in the classroom or engaging in anything else except sleep. In addition to keeping them physically inactive, commercial TV exposes them to violence, stereotyped sexual and racial attitudes, and an endless string of commercial messages. Limit their viewing hours and your children will rediscover their books, their friends, and their bicycles. You may want to set up a chart so that children can monitor the amount of time they watch television and then reward them for keeping their TV time between zero and ten hours a week.

Is it important to get my daughter the one thing she really wants? She's only three and a half, and she wants a Barbie doll.

Most of the child specialists we've talked with agree that getting your child that one thing that's at the top of her list helps her see that you are paying close attention to her wishes and dreams, even though—and this is the tricky part—you may not fully support them. But on the other hand, if you have *strong* objections to your children's requests, it's better to be honest and help them think of other things they'd like equally well. When older children ask for gifts that are too expensive, for example, it's better to say quite honestly, "That sounds like a great gift, but we can't afford it this year," than to give the gift along with the hidden message that you regret spending so much money on them.

My parents give my children far too many gifts. We only give them a few, but the total haul is way too much. How can I ask them to give fewer gifts without hurting their feelings?

When each well-meaning grandmother, grandfather, aunt, and uncle adds three or four gifts to the collection, children may have to spend hours opening them. And it's clear to everyone watching that a fraction of that number would be ultimately more satisfying. Quite a few of the parents we've talked with have found solutions to this problem; here are two of them:

Last year my mother asked us what our three-year-old wanted for Christmas. In the past she had given Melissa four or five presents. We suggested that Mother spend a day with her instead, because spending time with Grandma was the best present of all. So Melissa had a wonderful day at the zoo with her grandmother and grandfather while my wife and I had a free day together to work on Christmas gifts. It was perfect.

Two years ago we asked people to send us family gifts at Christmas and save individual presents for the kids' birthdays. It works beautifully. Now the boys get one present apiece from us, one from

Santa, and then games and books the whole family enjoys from everyone else. It takes the focus off each one of us and puts it on the family.

I don't feel comfortable telling other people how many gifts to give my children. Is there any other way to keep the total number of gifts under control?

Again, we turn to some wise parents for their solutions.

When relatives bring Christmas presents we let our children open them right away instead of letting them pile up until Christmas Day. Then the person who brought them gets to see the children's reaction. And if a present comes in the mail, we try to find a picture of the person who sent it to show to the kids as they're opening the package. They used to think the gifts came from the mailman.

When Michael was three years old, he was given over thirty presents for Christmas. We kept most of them stored away and brought them out one at a time later in the year. He still had ten presents to open on Christmas morning, which was more than enough.

How can I encourage my children to be more generous at Christmas? All they seem to think about is themselves.

Probably the best way to encourage generosity in your children at Christmas is to set a good example yourself. For example, let your children see how much fun you have giving gifts to other people. If you regularly make charitable donations at Christmas, tell them about it, and include their names in the gift. And make a special effort to give generously of your love and attention during the holiday season.

To more directly involve your children in being generous, you may wish to add special "giving" traditions to your celebration. That way, each holiday season teaches them more about the true meaning of Christmas. But be sure to make these projects fun for the children, and don't force the issue. A child's awareness of and concern for other people develops gradually over the years—and the most potent lessons come just from watching you.

Here are some ways other families around the country have set the stage for generosity:

In our family, my sisters and I become "secret friends" each Christmas. We draw names from a Christmas stocking and do neat things for that person, like washing dishes or helping find something that's lost. On Christmas Eve we exchange cards saying whose secret friend we've been.

We tell our four- and two-year-olds that Santa Claus not only brings gifts, but takes gifts that have been left for him under the tree to give to needy children. Last year our four-year-old son decided to leave his favorite truck for Santa, and he seemed to feel especially good about that.

Every Christmas I set aside a special day to take my daughter Christmas shopping to help me choose gifts for her cousins. We make it a leisurely day, go to a special restaurant for lunch, and talk about her cousins and what they would like. She comes up with wonderful ideas—things I never would have thought of.

My kids are really extraordinary in the amount of time and thought they give each other at Christmas. We've encouraged that by giving the kids a certain amount of money to buy gifts for their brothers and sisters, and the only rule is they have to cover everybody. By the time they are eight or nine, they see Christmas as a time to show each other they really do understand who they are, what they like, and what would make them happy.

Once a year I take my children grocery shopping and we fill up a sack with Christmas goodies—dates, candied fruits, nuts, butter, brown sugar, honey, all those expensive ingredients you have to buy at Christmastime —and then we leave them off at the Loaves and Fishes center to be given to a needy family.

How can I help my young children realize that Christmas is Jesus' birthday, not their own?

If yours is a Christian family, celebrating the birth of Jesus may be the primary source of your holiday joy, and while you may take part in Christmas activities at church, you also want to bring those spiritual insights home. Here are ways that other families have helped their children celebrate Jesus' birthday.

We hang eight stockings by the mantel, one for each of our seven children and one for Jesus. All of the kids write cards to put in Jesus' stocking, telling Him how they want to be next year.

We have a birthday party for Jesus. This is the family tradition that our children look forward to most of all.

*The
four things
children
really want
for
Christmas*
✳

In our family we bring out pieces of our family crèche a few at a time to correspond with the Christmas story. The week before Christmas, we bring out the stable, Joseph and Mary, and the animals, and let the children play with them. Every time I turn around they are in a different arrangement. On Christmas morning I bring out the Baby Jesus. And the wise men make their first appearance on Epiphany. This helps my children reenact the birth of Jesus and adds an element of drama to the crèche that it wouldn't have otherwise.

When our children were very young, we read them Luke after they opened their presents, and let them dress up with scarves, robes, and jewelry to playact the story of Jesus' birth.

The Gift of Time by Margaret E. Miller, Rev. Robert Miller, Loretta Vanderveen, and Carl Vanderveen (Wilton, Conn.: Morehouse-Barlow Company, 1977) is a resource book for Christian families "designed to bring into focus the true meaning of the Advent, Christmas, and Epiphany seasons and their relevance to family life." Through crafts, prayer, and simple skits, this book helps you make the entire holiday a spiritual experience for your family. Here's a quotation from the introduction to the book: "These seasons—ADVENT, CHRISTMAS, EPIPHANY—call out to us for silence and significance. They speak to us and to our children of becoming more like those who came to Jesus with only the gifts of their hearts, with only the thoughts of being present at a mystery, with only the desire to bow down in awe. This book is dedicated to the silence and awe and mystery of these seasons, and to family relationships given the power to grow in ritual, prayer, and togetherness of the celebrated seasons."

How can I help my children see that Christmas is a time of goodwill toward all people on earth?

Mankind's hopes for greater understanding among all the peoples of the world are resurrected each Christmas. But while this may be an idea that is dear to you, it can seem like a complex and difficult concept to communicate to your children—especially if all of your friends have more or less the same background and your winter travels are limited to trips to the grocery store.

But there are some practical ways to help your children become more aware of the other inhabitants of the world. Give Peace a Chance is a board game that introduces players to the language, methods, and some

71

of the heroes of peace. It promotes the concept that "we all win if there is world peace." The game is for two to four players, ages nine to adult and is produced by Peace Works, Inc. located in Fresno, California. For more information call (209) 435-8092.

To help your children understand other cultures, you might take advantage of the wonderful gifts available from UNICEF, the United Nations International Children's Emergency Fund. Each year the UNICEF winter catalogue features books, games, puzzles, and paper dolls that can help acquaint young children with their counterparts around the globe. The gifts are not only handsome and well made, but your check will go to help children in developing nations the world over. For information on alternative gift sources such as UNICEF and how to contact them, see pages 184–186.

And since peace begins at home, you might want to order your Christmas games from Family Pastimes, a Canadian business that designs games of cooperation rather than competition. Here's a comment from one of its customers: "It's strange to play a game, enjoy the evening, and have no family tensions." To order the catalogue, write to: Family Pastimes, R.R. 4, Perth, Ontario, Canada K7H 3C6; or phone (613) 267-4819.

What are some simple traditions that will keep my children from having to wait so long for Christmas to come and then feeling so disappointed when it's over?

Here are some suggestions from other parents on how to spread out the joy of the holiday season:

Last year I made a family calendar for the month of December and drew pictures on it showing when things were going to happen. I drew a tree on the day we were going to get the tree, airplanes on the days that Grandma and Grandpa were flying in and leaving, and a big birthday cake on December 29, which is my five-year-old's birthday. Both of my children looked at it a lot and seemed to get a lot of satisfaction out of knowing when things were going to take place.

To help my two preschool girls count down the days to Christmas, I make a "button banner" for them, an idea I got from the wonderful book *The Gift of Time* [see page 71]. The banner is made by cutting two eighteen-inch strips of three-inch-wide ribbon. On one strip of ribbon, I sew a string of eight large buttons spaced about two inches apart. On the other ribbon, I make eight buttonholes, with the exact same spacing. I place the two strips of ribbon together, sew them together at the top, and button the buttons. At the top of the banner I glue on a felt cutout of a bell. Each night starting on December 18, one of my two girls gets to unbutton a button as I read the following poem.

Button Banner Poem
December 18 to Christmas
Is the longest time of the year.
Seems that dear old Santa
Never will appear.

How many days till Christmas
It's mighty hard to count.
So this little button banner
Will tell the right amount.

Undo a button every night
When the sandman casts his spell.
Christmas Day will be here
By the time you reach the bell.

I always buy a jigsaw puzzle for the family to put together the day after Christmas. It keeps us all together doing something, but also gives us a quiet way to wind down.

We put a silver cup filled with red-hots on the Christmas tree, and these aren't to be eaten until we take down the tree. it's such a simple thing, but Megan really looks forward to it.

We celebrate each of the twelve days of Christmas with simple activities geared for our children. One day is Kids-Choose-the-Menu Day, another is Grandmother Day, and another is Hear-a-Story-As-Many-Times-As-You-Want Day. On the twelfth day of Christmas, we have an End of Christmas Ceremony and carefully pack away all the decorations. This puts an ending on the season and promises that it will come again.

What should I tell my children about Santa Claus?

We hear this particular question over and over again. Parents want to give their children a full measure of holiday joy—including the wonderment of a fat, jolly elf squeezing down a too-small chimney. But many parents are concerned about being caught lying to their kids, and others have serious doubts about the modern-day Santa's function—isn't he in reality the patron saint of department stores?

Child psychiatrists, parents, and even children themselves seem to be in a quandary over this one. One three-year-old told his mother to put up a SANTA GO AWAY sign on the front door on Christmas Eve. His mother explained that he didn't like the idea of a strange man tramping around *his* house in the middle of the night—not even if he was bearing gifts.

Of all the answers to the Santa Claus dilemma, the one that we like best of all comes from the yellowed, cracking pages of a December 1896 *Good Housekeeping* magazine.

> The problem, then, is before us: What shall we do with Santa Claus? The anxious mother questions, "Would you have me tell my children nothing about Santa Claus? Would you leave all that beautiful part out of our child's life?" By no manner of means.
> Tell the child the dear old stories of the good Saint as often as you please, but tell them invariably as myths, as fairy tales. Tell them from babyhood, when the literal story will be all he will understand, until he reaches the age when he can grasp the spiritual idea and slough the literal off. If the child is always told the myth of Santa Claus as a fairy tale, he will have all the childish joy and will have nothing to unlearn. You need not fear that he will lose the child's right to happiness in the story because of this way of presenting it. To a child of three, the spiritual is unintelligible and the tale will be a simple actuality; when he reaches the age of five or six, his mind will readjust it to an ideality.
> Tell the child the truth, by all means, but remember that for him, as for all children, some of the deepest truths lie in the realm of fairy tale.

I'm a grandfather and I feel that my grandchildren's Christmas is too overdone. The kids seem exhausted and jaded by the whole ordeal. What can I do to calm things down without stepping on my daughter's toes?

Grandparents have a special role to play in the lives of their grandchildren, never more so than at Christmas. You may not be able to control what happens at your daughter's house at Christmas, but you can spend extra time with the children on your own terms. You can make gifts with them, go on winter walks, read books to them, take them shopping, and give them some much appreciated one-on-one attention. When things seem a bit hectic at your daughter's house, you can reassure yourself that you have provided an oasis of calm.

In the middle of one of our workshops, a man began enumerating all the things that had bothered him about his family at their last Christmas reunion: His brother had been overly critical of his wife, his father had watched television during most of the family conversations, his mother's cheerfulness had verged on hysteria, and his sister's children had been out of control. He summed up his reaction to the holiday by saying, "I wouldn't mind spending Christmas with my family—if only they'd behave."

His last remark echoes the secret thoughts of a lot of people. While they look forward to seeing their families at Christmas, the reunion is never quite as good as they had hoped. All too often, there's something or someone that disappoints them. Instead of relaxing into a warm family celebration, they find themselves feeling judgmental or aloof, or nursing hurt feelings. And when Christmas is over, they realize that they've missed an important opportunity: There they were surrounded by all the people they really care about, but feelings of deep contentment just weren't there.

So far in this book, we've looked at Christmas from the point of view of each member of the family: the wife, husband, and child. In this chapter we'll explore what happens when all the relatives get together at the Christmas reunion. We've learned that when people have a better understanding of the inner workings of the family Christmas, they go to the reunion with more realistic expectations. And this helps them come closer to realizing the full promise of the celebration.

To begin with, let's take a look at a minor, but not insignificant, part of family gatherings, the physical logistics. As everyone knows, there's a lot of sheer work involved in assembling a large family in one place. The hosts have to spend days cleaning and decorating the house, changing beds, planning meals, stocking the pantry, and coordinating schedules. Meanwhile, the guests have to assemble all their gifts, take care of their animals, make financial and travel arrangements, pack all their suitcases, and secure their houses. These details always take more time and effort than people allow for, and as a family finally piles into a car the day before Christmas to travel down the interstate, it's not uncommon for tempers to be a little frayed.

Then, when everyone's finally gathered together, there are always some minor inconveniences. There's not enough hot water for all the showers, there's always a line at the bathroom, noisy children interrupt Grandpa's nap, teenagers stay up too late listening to rock music, intrepid joggers wake everyone up in the morning, and there's a constant mess in the kitchen.

When everything's going well—when people are getting along, everybody's healthy, and everyone's willing to compromise—these things hardly matter. In fact, they can add to the spirit of fun. There's a feeling of vitality in a house that's teeming with newborns, teenagers, middle-aged people, and grandparents. However, it helps for people to be mentally prepared for the realities of such a gathering, so that they can take the inevitable ups and downs in stride.

But there's more to the dynamics of a typical Christmas celebration than cold showers, loud rock music, and noisy children. Obviously, a more significant factor in everyone's enjoyment of Christmas is how individual family members relate to each other. To a large degree, this is determined by how well they interact the rest of the year. However, more than people realize, Christmas casts a bright light on family relationships—highlighting both their strengths and their weaknesses. Suddenly, both the good times and the bad times can seem more intense.

This power of Christmas to heighten our awareness comes from a subconscious wish we all have to belong to perfect families. This is an understandable longing. If our families were perfect, says an inner voice, then we would have a better chance for survival. We would be nurtured and loved and be able to withstand the inevitable pain and hardship of everyday life. We begrudgingly accept our families' imperfections from January to November, but when we flip the calendar to December, we yearn to be blessed—just this once, just at Christmas—with a perfect family.

But few families ever fully measure up. Whenever a door is opened on a family reunion, there will always be imperfect people, complicated relationships, and unfortunate circumstances. Even in the most loving and supportive families, there is always an undercurrent of mixed emotions; a casual remark or a habitual gesture may be all it takes to bring back a flood of memories. This is only natural. People who have a long and intimate history together invariably have complex reactions to each other. Freud could have filled a notebook sitting on a couch at a single Christmas reunion. Unless people give up their fantasy of an ideal family and emotionally prepare themselves for a houseful of relatives with all their strengths and weaknesses standing out in bold relief, they're going to be disappointed.

This was especially true for a thirty-two-year-old woman named Sarah, a loan officer in a large bank in an East Coast city. Sarah told us about how disappointed she was in her parents the Christmas they came to stay with her. For weeks she had been looking forward to their visit. She and her parents hadn't seen each other in two years, and as she drove to the airport to pick them up, all she could think about was how great it would be to see them. She was especially eager to show them her house. She and her husband had been working on it for months, and had remodeled the spare bedroom just in time for their visit.

When she picked out their familiar faces from the crowd, she ran up to them and gave them each a big hug. But shortly thereafter, she was awash with complex emotions. Her first unexpected reaction came when her father discovered that his new luggage had been slightly scratched on board the plane. All at once she remembered how upset he often got over trivial matters, and she felt her stomach start to tighten. Although her father's anger subsided in a few moments, Sarah still felt on edge. How could she have forgotten about his bad temper? And her anxiety was compounded by the fact that her mother kept going on and on about their new Hartmann luggage and how much it cost. Sarah had also forgotten how status conscious her mother was. For the first time she found herself worrying about how her mother was going to view their slightly run-down neighborhood. It was not a part of town that her parents would ever live in.

On the way home in the car, Sarah felt these confusing feelings subside somewhat as she and her parents caught up on each other's activities. They really were quite loving and charming people, despite their faults. But throughout the rest of their visit, she continued to be disappointed by them. They weren't as perfect as she wanted them to be. For one thing, there was more tension between her mother and father than she remembered. And some of their attitudes seemed narrow and unforgiving. She kept sitting in judgment on them. When the visit was over, she was glad that they had come, but she was equally relieved that they had left.

Like many people, Sarah had set her heart on her relatives' being larger than life, and it was only when she was face-to-face with them that she saw them as they really were. Then she had to confront her disappointments all over again. Instead of loving and accepting them as imperfect human beings, she found herself being overly critical. If she had made more of an effort to think about the things that had disappointed her about her parents in the past and accepted the fact that they had probably not changed, she could have marshaled her feelings of acceptance and felt less emotionally distant from them.

People from nontraditional families may need to make an even greater effort to accept their families as they really are. Everywhere they look, the two-parent, two-child family is glorified. Christmas commercials show both Mom and Dad trimming the tree while two pajama-clad kiddies help out. Magazine ads show Dad assembling a bicycle on Christmas Eve with Mom smiling in the background. Soft-drink commercials show a family piling into the car to go to Grandma's, with no stops along the way to drop assorted children off at their "real" mom's or dad's. It's always one big, happy, storybook family settling into a traditional celebration.

This ever-present image of the "perfect" family serves only to remind people in nontraditional families of what they don't have. The rest of the year they are given sympathetic support and specific advice on how to create a new, strong family identity. But at Christmas, the rug is pulled out from under them, and they are left alone to cope with their "imperfect" families.

Barbara, the single mother of two girls aged nine and eleven, told us that the first Christmas after her divorce was painfully hard. "I looked around me," she said, "and all I could see were happy couples. And my girls kept grieving for their father. They kept thinking, 'Poor Dad. All alone.' " Everything reminded Barbara and her children of what they had lost.

One of the things that often helps people like Barbara come to terms with their family circumstances is to realize that traditional families—with a homemaker mother, an employed father, and a couple of children—are in the minority. More than 50 percent of all women are employed outside the home. Over 20 percent of all children live with one parent.

When nontraditional families accept the fact that they, like millions of others, are not going to fit into a stereotyped mold, they can start building celebrations that work for them. The second Christmas after her divorce, Barbara was able to do this. She took another look around her and saw that she had more single friends than she thought. So she decided to invite a group of single women and their children to a three-day celebration. "It wasn't really a party," she said. "It was 'Come, be part of my family.' " She carried on her usual traditions with whoever was there. People felt free to sack out on the couch and raid the refrigerator, and the children had a three-day slumber party. She told us that everyone had a wonderful time. "We laughed until our sides ached," she said. "We were women survivors together."

We've met many families like Barbara's that have found ways to create rewarding Christmas celebrations. And whether they were rich or poor, large or small, whether they included two parents or one, they accepted their families for what they were and built on the solid foundation of their real strengths. In the following pages, you will find a few simple exercises that will help you gain new appreciation of your own family, and answers to the most common questions people have about their families at Christmas. The questions and answers concentrate on specific problems, such as how to cope as a single parent, how to handle excessive drinkers, how to ease the strain of a large family reunion, what to do if you are facing Christmas all alone, and how to enrich a small family gathering.

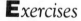

Exercises

THE PERFECT-FAMILY SYNDROME

No family is perfect, but if you can accept your family as it really is, you're going to have a more enjoyable celebration. This first exercise helps you take a look at your family members and explore your hidden expectations for them.

1 Write down the names of family members that you have complicated or mixed feelings about. Leave a blank space after each name.

2 After each name, write down something that troubles or disappoints you about that person.

Here's an example. Mary did this exercise and made the following comments about her family members:

Person	What I don't like
Dad	Drinks too much
Mom	Too uptight and busy
Louise	Overly talkative
Mark	Too withdrawn

3 If you have little reason to believe that people are going to change the characteristics that bother you, look again at each person's name and tell yourself, "I accept the fact that this person will probably ———," filling in the way that person will most likely behave.

Mary did this part of the exercise and told herself that she would try to accept the fact that her father often drank too much at Christmas. She realized that her mother chose to be so busy and that, even though any number of people offered to help her, she was determined to run the show. Her sister Louise had always talked too much and always would. And her brother Mark often backed away from the family, probably for the very reasons that she did. While she experienced some disappointment in realizing these things about her family, she felt clearheaded about what the visit would be like.

4 Now think of one thing that you especially like about each of the people on your list. Write those desirable qualities down by their names.

FAMILY STRENGTHS

When people are able to focus on their family strengths and not dwell on their weaknesses throughout the holiday season, they find that Christmas is many times more enjoyable. Whether you have specific family problems or not, this exercise will make you more aware of your family's strong points.

Read the following statements. When a statement is a family strength, mark it with a star. If it is a lesser strength, mark it with a check. Leave it blank if it does not describe your family at all.

✳ We have common spiritual beliefs or accept each other's different beliefs.

✳ We know how to have fun together.

✳ For the most part, we communicate with each other well.

✳ We openly express our love and affection.

✳ We have similar life-styles and values or accept each other's differences.

✳ We do not have serious money problems.

✳ We usually feel relaxed and comfortable around each other.

✳ We have common Christmas traditions or make a special effort to respect our differences.

✳ We have compatible styles of child rearing.

✳ We don't have serious alcohol problems.

✳ Other

(If you have few positive responses, make a special effort to fill in the "other" category.)

Questions and **A**nswers

Our Christmas is practically spoiled every year by an alcoholic family member. What should we do?

This is a very common problem. One out of every ten people in this country has a drinking problem. Chances are, when your family gathers at Christmas, one or more of them are struggling with alcoholism. At one workshop we gave for the parents of grade-school children, we asked the participants to think of a significant Christmas memory. Six out of the ten described unhappy experiences involving alcoholic parents.

When you stop to consider what happens at Christmas, this excessive drinking isn't surprising. Many of the pressures that people regulate successfully the rest of the year are intensified by the wish for a perfect Christmas, and drinking is an escape. Family members who may be uncomfortable or bored with each other take a shortcut to conviviality. Overworked parents look for a fast way to relax before the next round of holiday obligations. And the person alone finds he likes his own company better with each succeeding glass.

On top of this, everything about the secular holiday invites people to indulge themselves. Christmas has always been a festival of abundance, and drinking is one of its principal rituals. But the line between abundance and overabundance is a fine one. All you have to do is scan the December magazines to understand how subtle and all-pervasive this invitation to drink is. The message is clear: People who drink at Christmas are handsome, sexy, affluent, young, intelligent, and classy.

And then there is the Christmas office party. One man described the tradition this way: "Every year my business would host this enormous office party with an open bar on Christmas Eve. My wife would knock herself out doing something nice at home and the kids would be there waiting for me. Many times, I either didn't get home until late, or I came home drunk. The kids would have to be shushed away and apologized to, and the whole thing would be spoiled."

There is no denying that drinking is a problem for countless families at Christmas, but in order to understand this problem better, it's important to realize that not everyone who overdrinks at Christmas is an alcoholic. An alcoholic drinks excessively all year round, whether it is Christmas or not. A "simple excessive drinker" overdoes it on occasions like Christmas.

True alcoholism is a complex problem. Whatever cajoling or manipulating you do will most likely have no effect. One alcoholism counselor we talked with suggested not inviting people with a history of overdoing it to your Christmas festivities, and telling them plainly why. As he says, "Alcoholics are not fragile people."

If a member of your group is a newly recovered alcoholic (someone who's been sober for one year or less), he or she is vulnerable to the temptations of Christmas drinking. You can do yourself and that person a favor by either serving no alcoholic beverages, or making sure that nonalcoholic alternatives are available. In either case, it's important to treat a recovered alcoholic like a normal person by not making an issue of alcohol one way or the other. And, of course, *never* say to an alcoholic, "Come on, one drink won't hurt you." Although alcoholics know they cannot take even one drink without serious consequences, social pressure is something they don't need.

If you are confronting simple excessive drinkers at Christmas, you have more leverage. Again, straight honest talk about what you expect can be effective. But in addition, planning functions where alcohol is either absent or kept to a ritual minimum can help, even if that means that some people prefer not to accept your invitations.

Excessive drinkers usually like company and will often pressure the people around them to join in. Don't be afraid to say no even if doing so offends them. Because drinking is often a symptom of boredom and a replacement for genuine involvement with other people, you can also plan activities that get everyone physically active and involved in some way (see Chapter 9 for suggestions).

If you find *yourself* tempted to drink more than you know you should during the holidays, it might help to remember that alcohol is a depressant. If you are feeling a little down anyway, drinking is liable to make you feel worse. Physical activity and exercise, however, have the opposite effect. Cultivate some activity you enjoy that gets you up and moving about, and you may find that your alcohol intake slows down.

I come from a large family. We have so many family obligations that by the time Christmas is over, we're all exhausted. Is there a way to make our Christmas less hectic?

What can you do if your extended-family Christmas feels more like an Olympic marathon than the restful, revitalizing celebration you dream about? Although the answer will be different for every family, we have three suggestions that will help you get closer to your own solutions.

First, ask yourself why you feel exhausted and wrung out during Christmas. Are you trying to see too many people in too short a time? Is traveling the problem? Does your visiting schedule ignore the needs of young children? Or, while your schedule is reasonable, are your relationships characterized by conflict and tension? Or does a busy, crowded holiday simply run counter to your idea of what Christmas should be? Once you have identified the source of your uncomfortable feelings, you can start doing something about them.

Second, look for practical solutions, even if this means breaking with tradition. When people have a chance to pinpoint the pressures in their family celebrations, they usually see very quickly what they would like to do differently. Often they realize that what were once enjoyable traditions have become habits that no longer fit their changed circumstances.

One couple with four school-age children decided to make it a rule not to travel anywhere on Christmas Day. They stayed home, resolving to schedule family visits for other times. A couple with junior high schoolers had felt for a long time that they wanted to have Christmas in their own home before their children grew up and moved away. So they decided to invite the grandparents to visit *them* for a change on Christmas next year. And a woman who always felt exhausted at Christmas came to a better understanding of the stresses and strains of a yearly celebration involving her six brothers and sisters and their families. She decided to bow out of the next one and invite her favorite sister and her family for a New Year's visit instead.

Third, communicate your desires to your family. Even the thought of telling Grandma they won't be coming for Christmas gives some people the shivers. Although it isn't possible to make rules about how to approach all family members with changes in Christmas plans, here are some principles to keep in mind. Talk to people well ahead of time. Depending on the situation, you might want to broach the subject to several family members at once during a summer family reunion or at Thanksgiving, or you might decide that a private conversation, letter, or phone call well before Christmas is best. Also, be patient and don't expect to accomplish all the changes you hope for immediately. It can take some people a while to get used to the idea that Christmas isn't going to be the same forever. A seed planted this year could bear fruit next year. Most important of all, take the time to explain your feelings thoroughly and calmly, without blaming others or becoming defensive.

Many of the people in our workshops who have tried this direct, sensitive approach have had success. They say things like "It took my father a while to get used to the idea, but now he accepts it," or "As soon as my brother understood our reasons, he admitted that he was feeling the same way."

And frequently, such proposals are greeted with real enthusiasm and relief. It often happens that several people in a family are feeling the same need for change, and are only waiting for one brave soul to take a stand. A woman told us that a letter she had circulated to her five brothers and sisters suggesting a simpler Christmas opened dialogue with them on a deeper level than ever before.

I live alone and I'm worried about this Christmas. I won't be with my family and I haven't made any other plans.

More and more people in this country are living alone. The United States Census Bureau estimates that there were almost twenty-three million people living alone in this country in 1991. Many of them go home to extended families for Christmas, but an increasing number have no close family or, for a variety of reasons, decide not to rejoin their relatives during the holidays. Over the last few years, we have talked with a handful of single people who have chosen to spend Christmas alone. There are a number of things you can do alone that you cannot do as part of a family gathering. If spiritual experiences are important to you at Christmas, you can decide to spend time in prayer, meditation, or reading. You can spend time outdoors hiking, skiing, camping. You can play your favorite music for hours on end. You can eat when and what you want and generally set your own schedule.

One man, a hairdresser, told us that his job required so much day-to-day contact and conversation that he relished the idea of Christmas Eve and Christmas Day alone. When we asked him whether he did anything special, he told us that he saved up special reading material for these two days, prepared his favorite meal of fried shrimp for Christmas dinner, and put his favorite madrigal music on the stereo. Another woman we talked with made it a tradition to reserve her aunt's beach cabin for the few days surrounding Christmas. Because she was an artist and found the solitude of the ocean restful and refreshing, she viewed these few days as a great privilege. Her only nods to Christmas were a big fire in the fireplace, homemade eggnog, and the reading of Dylan Thomas's *A Child's Christmas in Wales* on Christmas Eve. But, as she hastened to tell us, when she got back to town, she also made it a tradition to balance her solitude by throwing a huge New Year's Eve party for everyone she knew.

Although there are some people who look forward to Christmas alone, the overwhelming majority like to celebrate with other people. If you want your celebration to be social, you will probably find that you have a lot of options. To some degree, whether you perceive your lack of family as an irretrievable loss or as a chance to explore new options depends on your attitude. Here are some suggestions to help you see the possibilities.

First, redefine your idea of "family." Most people think of family as a group of people fixed for them by the accidents of blood and marriage. Whether or not they like their brothers and sisters and aunts and uncles, there they are. But more and more people these days are picking and choosing the people they wish to spend Christmas with. They are rearranging themselves into groups held together by mutual goals and affection that function in the same relaxed, supportive ways as traditional families. You may know several unattached, compatible people who would welcome an opportunity to gather at your house and spend Christmas with you. This kind of "family by choice" gathering is common and accepted at Christmas these days.

Second, get involved in helping others. A lot of people are frustrated because they do not have the time or the flexibility at Christmas to do the charitable things that they would like. You have just such an opportunity. Several of the single people we have talked to have committed themselves to food drives, hospital and nursing home visits, or other selfless activities at Christmas and gotten immense pleasure from them. They found that it made them feel good to help other people, and that they helped themselves by gaining a broader perspective on their problems.

Third, allow yourself to respond to your own impulses. There is a wonderful freedom in being able to act on the spur of the moment. One man with no family told us that just before Christmas the previous year, he had split up with his girlfriend and moved to a new town. He found himself alone for the holidays. At first he was fearful, but he decided to trust himself and his resilience. On Christmas morning, he got the idea of making some banana bread and taking it around to his neighbors, whom he had not had a chance to meet. He told us that their reception of a strange man bearing slightly soggy, warm banana bread on Christmas Day was heartwarming. Even if they were in the middle of their own family activities, they stopped, asked him in for a drink, and got acquainted.

Fourth, accept invitations from families at Christmas. It's the rare family that hasn't, at one time or another, taken in an unattached person for Christmas. Far from being an intrusion, the new person becomes a positive factor in the celebration. These families not only enjoy the introduction of "new blood" into their gatherings, but also feel good about dispelling someone else's loneliness. When we ask people to tell us about their childhood Christmases, they often call up fond memories of a single person who spent Christmas with the family.

There is no reason single people can't have full, happy Christmases. If you know yourself well enough to know what you need, approach the holiday with a spirit of adventure and confidence, and do some advance planning, you will find that Christmas is a time you look forward to.

Our family is so small that I always feel something is missing at Christmas. What can we do to have a better celebration?

We are conditioned to think of a thirty-pound turkey roasting in the oven and fourteen dinner plates set around the extended dining-room table at Christmas. On some deep level, most of us want to be surrounded during our celebrations by a sea of smiling, familiar faces, made dear by the bonds of love and marriage. When we think of Christmas, we think of big families; it's a hard habit to break.

And we maintain this dream even though today's families are getting smaller. In 1991, the average number of people per household in the United States was 2.63. It's true that these small units can combine into larger family groups at Christmas and live out the American Christmas dream, but there are an increasing number of small families that spend Christmas by themselves. Either they don't have the money to travel, the distance is too great, or they are emotionally cut off from their larger families. Then they are left with the reality of a missing spouse, or too few grandparents, or not enough children or cousins or aunts and uncles at Christmas.

While some people adapt to a small Christmas just fine, others have trouble getting over the nagging feeling that something is wrong. If you find yourself feeling that your family isn't large enough, here are some suggestions.

Make an effort to appreciate all the advantages of a small family. Because there are so few of you, you avoid many of the problems that surface in large family gatherings. You don't have to take into account the preferences, moods, and habits of a large group of independent adults and their unpredictable offspring. You probably don't have to spend as much money or go to as much trouble to prepare for the holiday. And you have a greater chance of finding the peace and quiet that is so important for a deep enjoyment of the holiday.

When you take advantage of these pluses, new opportunities open up for you. One single woman told us about a refreshing change in her style of celebration. "It used to be just my mother, my father, and me sitting down to a big Christmas dinner and opening presents all by ourselves," she said. "Although we liked each other's company, there was this emptiness, and I kept wondering what else we could do. My father had the inspiration. He suggested that we go to a good restaurant for Christmas dinner instead, and spend a few days going to the best museums and galleries in Chicago. We had a wonderful time together."

You may also wish to include nonfamily members in your celebration. If you still feel that more is better, you can enlarge your definition of "family" by reaching out to nonrelatives and drawing them into your celebration. There are always people around who would appreciate an invitation to your Christmas dinner. There are charities to assist, nursing homes to visit, widowed friends to console, young people to mother, and other small families like yours that would appreciate more people around on Christmas Day.

Over the years, our workshop has been sponsored by a wide variety of organizations, including community colleges, churches, parents' groups, and social service agencies. But once, just once, it was offered as a "holiday event" in a large department store.

The irony did not escape us. There we were, offering our Unplug the Christmas Machine workshop in the throbbing heart of the Christmas Machine itself. Our workshop was held in a conference room on the tenth floor of the department store, the same floor as all the holiday gift wrap, Christmas cards, and decorations. And in order to get to the workshop, everyone had to file past the Designer Christmas Collection, an elegant display of old-fashioned rocking horses, Colonial Christmas tree ornaments, and eighty-dollar antique dolls. Stationed right outside our door was a twelve-foot-high Christmas tree made out of stuffed green satin triangles.

In good faith, we made some concessions to the department store. We changed the title of our workshop from Unplug the Christmas Machine to the more benign How to Have the Christmas You Really Want, and made a pact between us to focus our comments on how Christmas affects family life, rather than holiday commercialism. But we also made it clear to the coordinator of the event that when people are given the chance to examine their family celebrations in detail, they often decide to scale down their gift giving.

As it turned out, the people who came to this particular workshop were more upset than most about Christmas commercialism. The very first woman to speak said that she didn't enjoy buying gifts for four of the people on her gift list. They were all wealthy, and she could never figure out what to buy them. "No matter what I come up with," she said, "they can always go out and buy the next brand up the ladder. Christmas seems like an overabundance of things nobody wants or needs." The next person picked up her train of thought. "The only thing that seems to matter at Christmas is how much money you spend," he

※

Chapter six

INSIDE THE CHRISTMAS MACHINE

※

※

※

※

89

said. "It's pure economics. And when the spirituality leaves the holiday in favor of materialism, it leaves a very large hole." A third woman added, "I fret and fret about what to buy people for Christmas, but on Christmas Day, I'm always a little let down. Here I've spent months thinking of the perfect present—I have a file where I write down gift ideas all year long—and somebody looks at what I've given them for a minute, says, 'Thanks,' and puts it aside. Half of the time, I miss the mark." A fourth person said, "Or somebody gives *you* something that's way off target, and you do your best to cover up your disappointment. Gifts don't matter in the big picture—not for anybody but the kids. So why do we make them such a big deal? I don't understand it."

Later in the day, when we asked everyone in the group to create a fantasy of an ideal Christmas celebration, not one of the more than forty people in the workshop described a Christmas with elaborate gifts. In fact, if gifts were mentioned at all, they were simple handmade presents or intangible gifts like love and acceptance.

Even as these people were sharing their visions of a nonmaterialistic Christmas, a noisy crowd of shoppers just outside the room made it difficult to hear, so a man in the back of the room got up and closed the door. As he sat back down he said, "Here we are talking about cutting back on gifts in the city's largest department store at the height of the shopping season. I bet this is exactly what it felt like to be inside the Trojan horse."

No matter where we have given our workshop, what we have called it, or how little encouragement we have given people to talk about gift problems, there have always been a large number of people with mixed feelings about Christmas presents. Often, their positive and negative feelings run neck and neck. On the positive side, they like the fact that Christmas encourages them to reach out to family and friends. They get genuine pleasure out of giving presents to the special people in their lives. And many people like the fact that making or buying gifts exercises their creativity. It can be very satisfying to choose just the right gift for each individual or to lovingly craft presents. And there's yet another reason so many people enjoy holiday gift giving. When Christmas is over, everyone has presents to use and enjoy that serve as reminders of the people who gave them. The whole year can be made richer by the gifts exchanged at Christmas.

But despite these positive aspects, many people have problems with Christmas gift giving. While they are just as eager as anyone else to wish their family and friends a merry Christmas, they feel that the whole tradition has gotten out of hand. And when they stop to examine their gift giving habits, they realize that they have sincere and unselfish reasons for wanting to make changes.

For example, many people have problems with elaborate holiday gift giving for the simple reason that they can no longer afford it. A grandmother with five children and twelve grandchildren told us that when all her friends and relatives were totaled up, she was buying at least thirty gifts each Christmas. Before her husband had retired, this seasonal outpouring of love and generosity had been manageable. But now that they were living on Social Security, buying that many presents had become a financial burden. With each present she bought, she felt a twinge of anxiety: How were they going to come up with the money to pay for all those gifts?

Other people are unhappy with traditional holiday gift giving because exchanging typical consumer goods at Christmas has little value to them. It seems pointless to spend weeks struggling to think of novel gift ideas for relatives who have so many things already. These people would rather exchange simple handmade gifts, or spend the time and energy they would normally sink into Christmas presents just being with the people they care about.

Finally, many Christians are unhappy with the fact that the spiritual message of Christ has to compete with the want-me, buy-me message of the merchants. When they stop to think about the simple way Christ lived his life and his concern for "the least of these," celebrating his birth with a multibillion-dollar exchange of video games, popcorn poppers, designer jeans, sports equipment, and expensive adult toys seems strangely inappropriate. As one man said, "It's hard to see Christ in all the electric carving knives and shaving cream."

For these reasons and more, many people want to simplify their holiday gift giving to bring it more into line with their resources, values, and beliefs. While they want to give people symbols of their love and affection, they aren't convinced that the tradition has to be so expensive and elaborate.

Unfortunately, when people contemplate cutting back on their gifts, they run straight into a set of hidden gift-giving rules. Although few people are aware of it, an elaborate, unspoken code governs our seasonal exchange of gifts. These hidden rules help establish order in a complicated social ritual, but if they are adhered to religiously, they make it difficult to make any significant changes. What are these rules? Read through the following ten axioms and see if they ring a bell.

THE TEN HIDDEN GIFT-GIVING RULES

1 Give a gift to everyone you expect to get one from.

2 If someone gives you a gift unexpectedly, reciprocate that year. (Some people have prewrapped generic gifts set aside for just such an occasion.)

3 When you add a name to your gift list, give that person a gift every year thereafter.

4 The amount of money you spend on a gift determines how much you care about the recipient.

5 Gifts exchanged between adults should be roughly equal in value.

6 The presents you give someone should be fairly consistent in value over the years.

7 If you give a gift to a person in one category (for example a co-worker or neighbor), give a gift to everyone in that category, and these gifts should be similar in value.

8 Women should give gifts to their close women friends.

9 Men should *not* give gifts to their male friends—unless those gifts are alcoholic beverages.

10 Whenever the above rules cause you any difficulty, remedy the situation by buying more gifts.

While it is humorous to see these gift-giving conventions written down in black and white—and clearly, we have written some of them tongue in cheek—most people can remember times when they were tripped up by them. For example, a good friend of ours named Sharon told us about the following actual gift exchange, which grew increasingly complicated precisely because of these hidden rules.

Sharon's story started out simply enough. Her original intention was to give all of her friends baked goods for Christmas. But a problem came up when a friend named Meg told Sharon that she had found a "fabulous" gift for her. Sharon knew right away that the loaf of bread she had been

planning to give Meg would not match Meg's gift to her (*a potential
violation of Rule 5: Exchange gifts of equal value*), so she went out and
bought Meg a rather expensive present (*satisfying Rule 10: When in doubt,
spend more money*).

Sharon thought that this maneuver had resolved the dilemma, but
the situation grew more complex later that week, when Meg called to
say that their mutual friend Anne wanted to be there when they opened
gifts. This new development complicated matters because Sharon had
also been planning to give Anne simple baked goods for Christmas. But
now that Anne was going to be there, Sharon would have to get an
equally nice gift for her too (*or break Rule 7: Give similar gifts to people
in the same category*).

The actual gift opening turned out to be even more emotionally
difficult than Sharon had anticipated. Meg's gift to her was worth at
least twice as much as the one she had bought for Meg, despite her
efforts to even out the exchange (*breaking Rule 5 after all*). And Anne,
the innocent bystander, was visibly confused by the unexpectedly high
value of all the gifts. She gave both Meg and Sharon simple scarves and
was surprised to find herself caught in the middle of such an extravagant
gift exchange (*another violation of Rule 5*).

If the ten gift-giving rules were followed rigorously, there would be
no way to simplify gifts, because they lock everyone into a tit-for-tat
mentality and assure that each year's offerings will be at least equal to
last year's. But when people are determined to make their Christmas
presents more a genuine expression of their feelings and less a rule-bound
ritual, they can find ways to circumvent the hidden conventions. One
way for people to get around them is to openly declare their intentions.
Imagine how short and sweet Sharon's story would have been if she had
said to Meg at the outset, "It's very generous of you to buy me such an
expensive gift, but I only have a simple one for you."

Just being more aware of the gift-giving rules and how they further
or frustrate their goals gives many people the courage to do what they
really feel is best. For example, a woman named Sara told us that in
previous years she and her husband used to go through a convoluted
weighing and measuring with each present they gave. First they tried to
remember exactly what they had previously given certain people. Then
they thought about what those people had given them. Finally, they

tried to choose a gift that would be exactly equivalent to the one they thought they were going to receive. But the year after attending our workshop, she and her husband spent some time talking about gifts and decided to be less conscious of the rules. They decided to just pick out things that felt right to give and leave it at that. "We felt as if a weight had been lifted from us," she said.

Some people get around the restrictive gift-giving rules by getting together with family and friends to invent new ones. For example, one family from Oregon agreed to violate Rule 6 (gifts should be consistent from year to year) by giving each other explicit permission to vary the gifts. They decided to do this because they rarely had the same amount of time or energy to spend on gifts from year to year, making it hard to maintain a set standard. "Now if we're short of money or time, we just give what we comfortably can without having to apologize or feel guilty," said one of the family members. "I don't think any one of us could have felt this freedom without our getting together to talk about it."

Other families have agreed to deescalate gift giving by giving each other token presents, rewriting Rule 4 (gifts must be an exact measure of your regard for the recipient). One such family has started a tradition of buying gifts at garage sales. While secondhand gifts may offend some people, everyone in this particular family loves them. "We're all good scroungers," explained the mother. "And none of us has much money. So we prowl around secondhand stores and garage sales looking for things." Because the members of this family don't build up hopes for expensive, shiny new gifts, they approach the family gift exchange with a spirit of fun and humor. "Other people probably think we're strange," said a teenage daughter. "But we all look forward to opening our gifts and usually end up in hysterical laughter."

To some people, giving gifts of their time and energy seems a more genuine way to show affection than giving the usual store-bought gifts. For example, a fifty-year-old farmwife named Merrily wrote us a letter telling us that her family's gift to her was a "year of Wednesdays." She explained that her husband and daughter had volunteered to do all her household and farm chores each Wednesday, provided she used that time for creative pursuits. For over twenty years, she had been running the household and managing the family farm, filling in her few remaining hours with civic duties. Now, she told us, she was gratefully using this gift of time to take calligraphy lessons, practice the piano, write, and paint.

One couple learned that *not* giving *any* gift to one of their sons turned out to be the best gift of all. Joan told us that for years her son Peter had been telling her not to get him anything special for Christmas because he didn't need material things. But she and her husband had ignored his request because they didn't feel that they had any other way to relate to him at Christmas. Besides, they would have felt funny about giving a gift to one son and not the other. "So we always got Peter something," Joan explained, "and he would be polite about receiving it."

One year, she and her husband spent some time thinking about what their son was really trying to tell them. As a result, they decided to take the money they would have spent on Peter and donate it to a friend of the family who was a kidney dialysis patient. "We told Peter about it the week before Christmas," Joan said, "and he felt really good about it. It gave him a deep sense of pleasure to think that the money was going to help a family friend."

When people choose their gifts with love and sensitivity, not with an eye to the rules, the holiday takes on fresh meaning. What everyone wants from Christmas is an exchange of genuine love and goodwill, not a swap of material goods. Some people find that a traditional gift exchange gives them the feelings they're looking for, but others feel the need to create new traditions. In the following exercises, you will have a chance to clarify your feelings about gift giving. Then you can read answers to the questions we hear most often about gifts. In the Appendix there are specific gift-giving suggestions.

Exercises

GIFT INVENTORY
List all the people you gave gifts to last year. Be sure to include friends, neighbors, co-workers, and children of friends or neighbors. Put a dollar sign by each person you spent more than ten dollars on.

FOUR GIFT FANTASIES

1 Imagine yourself in the following situations and check the ones that are most appealing to you.

a You open the mail one morning and discover that you have inherited five hundred dollars to spend on Christmas presents this year.

b You are given two weeks of absolutely free time to devote to making Christmas gifts.

c Every member of your family is excited about exchanging simpler and less expensive gifts.

d Everyone in the nation decides to eliminate gift giving from the celebration. There is no holiday advertising, no gift-giving obligations. People celebrate Christmas by joining with family and friends, by feasting, and with family and community Christmas activities.

2 Judging by your reactions to these imaginary situations, what changes, if any, would you like to make in your family gift giving?

GIFT MEMORIES

1 Think back over past Christmases and remember a gift that you received that gave you great pleasure. What did you especially like about that gift?

2 Now remember a gift you received that made you feel anxious, confused, angry, or disappointed. What was it about that situation that bothered you?

3 All in all, what kind of gifts do you feel best about receiving and giving?

Questions and Answers

I'd like to simplify my gift giving but I'm not sure about the reaction of my family and friends. What should I do?

It can seem difficult at first to change entrenched gift-giving habits. You may be exchanging gifts with ten, twenty, or thirty people, and they probably have a wide range of values and feelings about Christmas presents. But if *you* feel that your gift giving has gotten out of hand, chances are many of the others do, too. Some of the people on your list may actually prefer making a special effort to get together with you during the holiday season in place of exchanging gifts, and others may find it a relief to give fewer or simpler presents. And the only way to find out is by talking with them.

But first, it might help you to get a better idea of which people on your list would be most receptive to simplifying gifts, and then to do some more thinking about alternatives.

Here is an exercise to help you survey your gift list. Look back at Exercise 1 and place a check mark by the name of any person on the list who you think might welcome an invitation not to exchange gifts. (They might be distant relatives or casual acquaintances who would find it a relief not to exchange gifts. On the other hand, they might be very good friends or close relatives who would prefer another way of making contact at Christmas.) Put a plus sign by anyone who you think might be willing to talk about exchanging fewer or simpler gifts. Put an X by anyone who you think would be opposed to any change whatsoever.

Now you have a better idea of how many people might be willing to explore gift-giving options. But what kinds of changes do you want to suggest? Here, we have listed the five most common gift-giving alternatives. All of them work well for some families. Read through them and check the ones that seem most suitable for yours.

1 Name drawing Put the family names in a hat and draw the name of one person to buy or make a gift for.

2 Trimming a few names Talk with the people who you think might welcome an invitation not to exchange gifts.

3 Family gifts Give one gift per household instead of a gift for each separate individual.

4 Just for kids Keep giving presents to young children only.

5 Alternative gifts Give simple handmade gifts or gifts of service; or spend your money on a special trip or vacation together.

Keep in mind that you don't have to find one alternative that works for everyone. You can make separate arrangements with each household.

Once you have a better idea of the kind of change you want to propose, you will want to talk with your friends and family as early in the year as possible. Many people like to get their gift buying out of the way early in the fall. If it's too late *this* year to make new arrangements, get together now to talk about what you want to do next year. (Doing this a year ahead of time is actually an ideal arrangement, because you will be talking about what you like and don't like about gift giving while the whole experience is fresh in your mind, and you will have a whole year to adjust to any changes.)

When you talk with your family and friends, keep five points in mind. (1) Choose a relaxed and comfortable time when people are in an accepting mood. (2) Be clear about your reasons for wanting to make changes. (3) Be open to other people's opinions and suggestions. (4) Keep in mind that other people probably have done less thinking about gifts than you have and want some time to consider before they come to any conclusions. (5) Don't be afraid to experiment. You might want to try out an alternative gift giving arrangement for a year and see how it works, then make some changes the following year.

We have learned that there can be an important side benefit to talking with your family about gift alternatives. Many people have told us that they had made better contact with their friends and relatives by getting together to talk about gifts than they had in years. It gave them a chance to share their good feelings about each other and become better acquainted with each other's values. And whatever their ultimate gift-giving decisions, they found that they were drawn closer together.

One large, extended family—the Andersons—told us how they simplified their gift giving, a story that illustrates many of the five points. After reading our book, one of the Andersons suggested that the adults simplify their gift giving by drawing names from a hat. That first year, however, none of the other family members was interested in making a change. Christmas had little meaning to them other than getting together, having a festive meal, and exchanging presents. Reducing the number of gifts felt like too big a sacrifice.

The next year, the sixty-six-year-old matriarch of the clan warmed to the idea of the name drawing. She and her husband were recently retired, so it was difficult for them to buy expensive gifts for their five adult children, their spouses, and ten grandchildren year after year. Understanding her plight, the rest of the family decided to give the name drawing a one-year trial.

The first year of the name drawing, there were many fewer gifts under the tree, and several of the adults acknowledged feeling a little disappointed; Christmas seemed anticlimactic. Nonetheless, the group decided to go ahead and draw names again.

The second year, people felt much more comfortable with the name drawing. They were already accustomed to having fewer gifts to open, and they were beginning to enjoy the luxury of having just one person to think about each year. It made buying or making that one gift all the more special.

An added benefit was the fact that the men were becoming more involved in Christmas. Before, their wives had done virtually all of the shopping and wrapping. Now each adult was responsible for getting a gift for one other person, which gave the men a chance to share the work load and exercise their creativity as well.

By now, the Andersons have been drawing names at Christmas for six years, and they embrace the new ritual wholeheartedly. It feels right to them to shift some of the focus from the gift giving to the sheer joy of getting together. Even the grandchildren have gotten into the act. Seeing how much fun the adults have with the simplified gift giving, they asked if they could have their own name drawing. Now each grandchild makes or buys a gift for a cousin.

What impressed us about this story is the fact that changing a long established Christmas tradition can take time. As in the Anderson family, some people may need to adjust to the idea of making a change before they can act. Then they need more time to adjust to the change itself. But people who embark on this process of change usually discover that it is well worth the effort.

I would like to make all my gifts, but I never have enough time. What should I do?

Handmade gifts seem like ideal Christmas presents to many people. They are more personal, less expensive, and often more satisfying to both the giver and the receiver. In fact, handmade gifts are so welcome at Christmas that many people feel they *should* make their gifts even when they don't have the time, talent, or internal motivation. Before you try to squeeze hours of gift making into your busy life, stop and honestly examine your feelings. If you find that you enjoy making gifts and they have high priority for you, turn to the Appendix and look for especially quick and easy homemade gift ideas.

I've felt uncomfortable opening gifts as long as I can remember. Why is that?

You have a lot of company. Most adults discover that they get more pleasure out of giving presents than receiving them. One reason you feel anxious opening gifts may be that it makes you feel as if you're onstage. Like most people, you probably feel the need to act pleased no matter what you find in the package, because you don't want to hurt anyone's feelings.

Another reason for your discomfort may be that you have hidden wishes that are not being fulfilled. It's very common for people to secretly wish for special gifts from their spouses or parents that show exactly how much they care. While the dreamers may know that this is unrealistic (the gift givers may be poor at choosing presents, or have very little time or money to devote to gift giving), they still harbor the wish.

Finally, you may be reacting to the fact that many gifts carry hidden messages. An example would be a husband's gift of a too small, slinky dress to his overweight wife. Gift giving is a complex social phenomenon that puts the relationships between individuals into tangible form, and the messages hidden in the gifts are often as complicated as the relationships.

My husband and I have very different ideas on gift giving. How can we come to see eye to eye?

You and your husband each have a long and complicated history involving Christmas presents, and as with most people, your past experiences with gifts are probably a determining factor in your present attitudes. One woman told us that gifts were not very important to her but her husband went overboard with them each Christmas. She couldn't understand this until he told her about his childhood celebrations. When he was young, he had often felt shortchanged by his family at Christmas. His brother and sisters always seemed to get the better gifts. As an adult, he wanted to make sure other people didn't feel slighted. You may find that if you and your husband shared some of your earlier associations with gifts, you would understand each other better.

On the other hand, your problem may be one of differing values, not different Christmas histories. If this is the case, sit down and share your opinions. Be prepared for some strong emotions. Many people have intense feelings about what role gifts should play in the celebration. You may find it easier to accommodate the other person's point of view once you understand the sincere feelings behind it. Finally, you may need to work out a compromise. For example, you may decide to let each spouse take responsibility for giving gifts to his or her own family members, or work out a balance between your points of view.

Rose is a tax accountant and the fifty-year-old mother of two teenage children. She told us that no matter how much energy she puts into Christmas, she often feels disappointed by the celebration. "I don't know if it's regret over what might have been, or memories of what used to be—all I know is that in recent years, Christmas has seemed rather pointless," she said. "When you take away the fuss and the bother, Christmas is just another big meal."

This is a common complaint. Many people tell us that they have a vague feeling of emptiness at Christmas. Even though they are doing things they have looked forward to all year long and are surrounded by their favorite friends and relatives, they still have the feeling that something is missing. For some reason, the vivid reds and greens of the holiday season merge into gray, and they find themselves just going through the motions of rejoicing.

At first, some people have a hard time explaining exactly what's wrong with Christmas because on the surface everything looks fine. But when they take a closer look, many of them realize that their celebrations lack depth and meaning. It's not enough that Christmas resemble a family birthday party or the biggest social event of the year. They want to be moved by the celebration. When they decorate, they want the result to be more than a beautiful house. They want to look around them and be filled with an air of expectancy. When they write a check to a charity, they don't want to be mentally computing the tax deduction. They want to be filled with genuine compassion for the people they are helping. And when they attend a worship service, they don't want to be just passive consumers of an hour's religious entertainment. They want to be filled with the spirit of God. At Christmas people want to reach down inside themselves and come up with feelings that are better, bigger, more joyful, more loving, and more lasting than their everyday ones.

But as the following workshop conversation shows, many people go through Christmas without this deep sense of joy.

First woman: You know, something I'm just beginning to realize is how self-centered my Christmas has become. Here I am talking about how my house looks and what other people think of me. I'm not reaching out, not doing things for people who don't have all that I do.

First man: Well, in our family, we do a few charitable things. But most of them are pretty mechanical. Pleas for money come in the mail and I write out checks. But I'm not really involved in any of the causes. I just save myself the guilt.

Second woman: I get to feeling very guilty at this time of year because we are not associated with a church. I think we should be more spiritual at Christmas. Both my husband and I went to Sunday school as kids, but we haven't raised our kids that way. Christmas is a church holiday. I feel my family is missing something.

Third woman: I'm Christian. And I go to the candlelight service on Christmas Eve. That's where Christmas comes alive for me. But on Christmas Day—when there are thirty-five people jammed together eating too much and giving presents that nobody needs—that's not Christmas. There's a big spiritual hole there.

Second man: I know what you mean. We go to church and have Advent ceremonies at home. But Christmas Eve and Christmas Day are totally irreligious. I think this adds to my feeling of emptiness. The spiritual message isn't there when it should be.

As these remarks show, both Christians and non-Christians can feel a spiritual emptiness at Christmas. Although the celebration has a fundamental religious significance for Christians, they must find a way to make these beliefs come alive. In a broad sense, both Christians and non-Christians are asking the same questions: How can Christmas connect me with ideas and experiences larger than myself? How can I share my blessings with other people? How can the celebration make me feel most whole and happy?

When people don't find satisfactory answers to these questions, some take it as a personal failure. What's wrong with *me* that I don't feel loving and generous and closer to God? Why haven't I felt even one moment of pure happiness? When they look around them, they see that others seem to have all the joy that eludes them, and they often feel alone in their disappointment. Then there are people who look outside themselves for the source of their discontent. Many blame Christmas commercialism. To them, the constant emphasis on the buying and selling of holiday happiness robs the celebration of its significance. They wonder if it's even possible to have a value-centered holiday when so many forces conspire against them. Other people attribute their lukewarm feelings to the idea that Christmas is basically a children's holiday and they've gotten too old to enjoy it. They look back nostalgically to their childhood Christmases and try to accept that those moments of joy are all in the past.

But for most people, the real problem with Christmas isn't that they are spiritually bankrupt or that Christmas is devoid of meaning. It's simply that they haven't taken the time to define for themselves what's most important to them about Christmas.

A lot of people go through the holiday season without a clear sense of what they value. While they have planned the details of their celebrations right down to the kind of cranberry sauce to serve at Christmas dinner, they haven't stopped to ask themselves the all-important question: Why am I celebrating Christmas? They rely on habit, other people's priorities, commercial pressures, or random events to determine the quality of their celebrations. But this is rarely successful. People need to make conscious choices because Christmas offers them so many possibilities. It's a time to celebrate the birth of Christ, the pleasures of family life, the importance of friendship, the delight of creating a beautiful home environment, the need for world peace, the desire to be charitable, and a host of other important values. When people don't sort out which of these ideas is most important to them, the celebration can seem fractured and superficial.

But choosing among all the rich possibilities of Christmas is not always easy. Often, people must choose between activities of seemingly equal value. For example, they must decide whether to spend their limited funds to buy more gifts for family and friends, or to make a contribution to an important charity. They must weigh the value of having a quiet, relaxed celebration against that of entertaining special friends. And if they are Christians, they must ask themselves what's more important, working for the church or spending more time with their families.

When people haven't resolved these larger issues, they find it hard to make the dozens of small decisions that confront them every day of the holiday season. For example, Louise, a young woman in her late twenties, told us about a puzzling experience she had had the year before. In the weeks just before Christmas, her mother had been feeling a little glum, and Louise decided that buying her mother an early Christmas present—something a little extravagant that she wouldn't buy for herself—might cheer her up. Louise deliberated on what to buy her mother for several days, and finally settled on a print that she had seen in an art studio.

One rainy afternoon right before Christmas, Louise left work to buy the print. On the way, she turned on her car radio and heard the announcer make a plea for more toy donations to the local charity drive. He said that the demand for children's gifts was much greater than expected, and that many children would go without toys unless people responded immediately.

Louise pulled the car over to the side of the road and sat there for a few minutes thinking about the announcement. How could she spend fifty dollars on an extra present for her mother when there were children facing Christmas without any toys at all? She decided that she couldn't buy the print after all. So she turned around and drove back home.

But the confusing thing to Louise was that she never donated the money to the toy drive. "I didn't do anything," she said. "I just went home and tried to forget about the print." Louise wanted to do something nice for her mother, but she felt guilty about spending so much extra money on someone who was comfortable already. And she wanted to help the children, but she wasn't clear enough about her priorities to actually go ahead and make the donation.

Like Louise, many people are so overwhelmed by the competing possibilities of the celebration that they find themselves unable to make any choices at all. And they often end up feeling guilty or disappointed by their inactivity. But other people have the opposite reaction. They see value in a wide range of holiday activities, and because they are energetic and resourceful, they try to squeeze them all in. These are the people who lead the community charity drive, make all their own tree ornaments from recycled objects, put on Christmas parties for the neighborhood children, make cookies for nursing homes, sew matching outfits for their nieces and nephews, and direct the church Christmas program. They want to do it all. Unfortunately, their pleasure in all these activities diminishes with each new one that's added. And they end up feeling numb and tired, cut off from the deep satisfaction they hoped all this effort would bring them.

Other people make the wrong choices. They don't do too little or too much; they simply put their time and energy into activities and projects that aren't right for them. For example, most people put a lot of time, money, and energy into gift giving. But when they sit down and sort out their values, many realize that spending time with their families, giving money to charity, or nurturing their spiritual lives— some other part of the celebration—is more important to them. For years they've been channeling the bulk of their resources into a part of Christmas that has only limited value to them, and still they wonder why the celebration seems so shallow and meaningless.

It's clear that being unsure of their values is the source of many people's unhappiness at Christmas. But we've been encouraged by how quickly and easily people can decide what's most important to them. All they need to do is to become more aware of the need to make choices, have some sense of what those choices are, and set aside a little time to reflect on them. With just a few minutes of prayer, meditation, or conscious decision making, most people gain a much better sense of how Christmas should be. At the end of this chapter we've included an exercise that will help you take a look at all the values that are competing for your attention at Christmas and rank them in order of priority. This simple exercise may be all you need to gain a better understanding of what's most important to you during the holiday season.

We had a demonstration of how quickly this can happen when we were at a radio station talking with a man who was about to interview us on a talk show. Just before we went on the air, we handed him a copy of the values exercise that's at the back of this chapter. Even though we were scheduled to go on the air in just two minutes, he was intrigued by the exercise and decided to see how much of it he could complete. In that short amount of time, he was able to identify one of his major problems with Christmas: He wasn't spending enough time with his kids. His children's happiness was his top priority, but he had allowed a lot of other things come first. He resolved to go home and talk with his wife about cutting out some of their social obligations so he could spend more quiet evenings at home with his family.

Like this radio announcer, many people decide to make some adjustments in their holiday plans once they have a clear sense of what's important to them. For example, they may decide to cut back on other activities in order to spend more time with their families, or they may decide to help out with a charity drive so they can translate their generous impulses into action.

This self-knowledge also helps people make the dozens of smaller, spontaneous decisions that can invest the entire holiday season with special meaning. In the case of Jim, a salesman and the father of three children, a keen awareness of his values enabled him to make a spur-of-the-moment decision that made all the difference in his appreciation of the holiday.

In early December, when Jim was driving his family home from a school crafts fair, he stopped the car so a bent old man could cross the street. Jim watched the man's slow progress for a moment and then made a quick decision. Without saying a word he pulled the car over to the curb, reached for a package of cookies he had bought at the fair, jumped out of the car, and ran after the old man.

As Jim overtook him, the old man became alarmed. He wheeled around and drew back his fist, as if trying to defend himself. Jim quickly said that he wasn't going to hurt him. When the man realized that Jim had something to give him, his eyes filled with tears and he asked Jim why he was giving him a present. Jim was surprised to hear himself say, "Because it's Christmas and I love you." As the old man accepted the cookies, Jim felt tears coming to his eyes too. "I was overcome with emotion for this stranger," he told us. "That moment captured the true meaning of Christmas for me."

Jim learned that a spontaneous act of generosity to a stranger was what he needed in order to feel more spiritually alive at Christmas. Although this kind of encounter wouldn't be satisfying to everyone, many of the people we talk to say that they feel better about Christmas when they find some way to reach out to others. The challenge is to learn which avenues of expression are most likely to give them the satisfaction they are looking for. Some people feel comfortable writing a check to a favorite charity, while others show their concern by spending time with a sick friend or a lonely relative. People have their own ways of reaching spiritual fulfillment.

Most people find satisfaction at Christmas in traditional ways. They come to feel connected to other people by celebrating with family and friends, get spiritual fulfillment from going to church, and express their generosity and goodwill by donating money to charities and exchanging gifts. These traditions connect them to past Christmases, to other people, and to important ideas and values. And they give them a sense of identity and harmony as well as pleasure.

But we've been surprised at how many people get spiritual rewards at Christmas in highly individual ways. For example, a friend of ours said that his most meaningful Christmas had been spent in the mountains with his wife. A middle-aged woman told us that she had enjoyed Christmas most the year she attended the Christmas services of three different denominations, discovering the common themes in all the sermons. And a woman that we met at a conference told us that she had found the feeling of family she was looking for by adopting an old woman in a nursing home as her children's grandmother and inviting her into their home every Christmas.

It's important to realize that many of the rare moments of joy that light up the holiday cannot be programmed or prescribed. They come as gifts. An unexpected phone call from someone you love, a child's heartfelt generosity, the spontaneous happiness that comes over you in a room smelling of evergreens and glowing with candles, a fresh Christmas snowfall, a feeling of harmony with the world around you—these things cannot be manufactured. But when people are clear about their values and find meaningful ways to express them, they've laid the foundations of a soul-satisfying celebration.

In the pages that follow, you will find a values exercise that will help you clarify what's most important to you at Christmas. And then you can read answers to some specific questions people have about expressing their values.

Exercise

WHAT ARE YOU CELEBRATING?

In general, people ask Christmas to do too many things for them. They want it to strengthen their family bonds, give their spirits a lift in the dark days of winter, stimulate their compassion and generosity, help them keep tabs on far-flung friends, confirm their deepest religious beliefs, show off their skills as hosts and hostesses, establish their rank in the social order . . . the list goes on and on. No one celebration can do it all.

This values-clarification exercise will help you decide which parts of Christmas are most deserving of your efforts. Once you have decided that, you will be able to plan a celebration that is in harmony with your deepest beliefs and most expressive of who you are as an individual.

As you do this exercise, keep in mind that there are no "right" or "wrong" values. This has been brought home to us time and time again in the many opportunities we have had to conduct our Christmas workshop. During a workshop that we gave to a group of fifty people in Seattle, we read the list of ten values and asked people to raise their hands when we mentioned the one that was most important to them. As is often the case, there was a big show of hands for the second value—spending time with the family—and the fourth value—celebrating the birth of Christ. When we got to the fifth value—gift giving—only one person raised her hand, a petite woman in her seventies. A Franciscan nun, she told us she saw Christmas not as a time to celebrate the birth of Jesus—something she did every day of her life —but as a time to make gifts for her family and friends who were scattered around the world.

During another workshop, an active church leader told the group that her highest value at Christmas was finding time to be relaxed and renewed. "I am so busy throughout the year," she said, "that I long for those few weeks of vacation. I don't volunteer at church. I don't volunteer at school. I just stay home, enjoy my family, and rest. I love it."

There are no right and wrong answers. No "shoulds." The message of this exercise is that Christmas is rich in meaning, and you need to decide what is most important to you in order to have the most satisfying holiday season.

To complete the exercise, read through the following ten value statements, cross off those that have no importance to you, and add any equally important ones that we have not included. Then decide which of the remaining values is most important to you. Put a "1" beside that sentence. Then find the one that is next important to you and put a "2" beside it. Continue in this manner until each statement has been assigned a different number. Even a value that has a low priority can still be important to you. Remember: 1 is highest and 10 is lowest.

✳ Christmas is a time to be a peacemaker, within my family and the world at large.

✳ Christmas is a time to enjoy being with my immediate family.

✳ Christmas is a time to create a beautiful home environment.

✳ Christmas is a time to celebrate the birth of Christ.

✳ Christmas is a time to exchange gifts with my family and friends.

✳ Christmas is a time for parties, entertaining, and visits with friends.

✳ Christmas is a time to help those who are less fortunate.

✳ Christmas is a time to strengthen bonds with my relatives.

✳ Christmas is a time to strengthen my church community.

✳ Christmas is a time to be relaxed and renewed.

Questions and **A**nswers

The most important thing to me about Christmas is its promise of peace on earth. What can I do at this time of year to further the cause of world peace?

An increasing number of people are looking for ways to make "Peace on Earth, Goodwill Toward Men" more than just a message on their annual Christmas cards. One way to act on your concern is to redirect some of the money you've set aside for holiday expenses to a peace organization. You could make a donation, subscribe to a peace newsletter or magazine, volunteer your time, or give a gift donation or subscription. If you are a member of a church, your denomination undoubtedly has its own peace program. Or you may want to contribute to a national organization. Here are some of the best-known groups:

American Friends Service Committee (AFSC)

Founded in 1917 by the Society of Friends, AFSC tries to encourage and support human survival by working for the abolition of war. In order to achieve this goal, it seeks a nonviolent world order based on global justice and a more equitable sharing of the world's resources. To make a donation or to volunteer your time, write to: The American Friends Service Committee, 1501 Cherry Street, Philadelphia, PA 19102.

Fellowship of Reconciliation (FOR)

"FOR is a company of men and women who have a vision of and a commitment to the creation of a peaceful, just world community with full dignity and freedom for every human being." FOR was organized in England in 1914 when an English Quaker and a German Lutheran pastor pledged to remain friends and continue to work for peace, even though their countries were at war. While most of the members of FOR are Christians, the participation of people of Jewish faith and other religious traditions is encouraged. If you would like to make a Christmas contribution to FOR, send a check to: FOR, P.O. Box 271, Nyack, NY 10960. FOR publishes a magazine called *Fellowship* eight times a year that keeps readers informed of ongoing peace activities and contains thought-provoking articles on issues relating to peace. A subscription is fifteen dollars.

Beyond War

Beyond War is a nonpartisan, educational movement whose stated goal is "to assure that the genius of the human species and the resources of the planet are used for the benefit of life." Beyond War focuses on what it calls the following basic realities: (1) All life is interdependent and interconnected. (2) Diversity is desirable and is to be understood and encouraged. (3) All conflicts can and must be resolved without resorting to violence or war.

Your financial support is welcome. A contribution of twenty-five dollars entitles you to a one-year subscription to its monthly publication, *On Beyond War*. Write to: Beyond War, 222 High Street, Palo Alto, CA 94301. Phone: (415) 328-7756. Fax: (415) 328-7785.

I feel strongly that I have an obligation to my church at Christmas, but so often I get stretched too thin. I end up feeling exhausted and depleted instead of renewed by my obligations. What can I do?

Because we talk with so many committed church people about Christmas, we know how common the problem of burnout is. It seems almost axiomatic that a few capable, energetic people carry most of the responsibility of church activities. As one church leader told us, "If you want to get something done, ask someone who is already busy."

The first step in getting control of your church commitments during November and December is to sit down with a blank piece of paper and a calendar and try to get a good idea of how busy you are likely to be. Write on the calendar any non-Christmas church activities that will probably occur during the season (include regular committee meetings, social events, children's activities, and so on). If you don't know the dates, write the items on the piece of paper under the heading "Ongoing Church Commitments." Next, write down any work or social commitments that you know about (include dinner meetings, out-of-town trips, bridge groups). If you don't know when they will occur, put them under the heading "Work and Social Commitments." Finally, do the same for your family Christmas activities. Although many of these activities will be hard to place on the calendar (such as baking cookies with the kids, mailing packages, shopping for special groceries), try to pin down as many of them as possible on specific days. The rest can go on your paper under the heading "Family Activities." At this point, you will have a pretty good idea of what your schedule will look like this holiday season, and you will know how many other church responsibilities you can comfortably take on.

The second step is to determine what obligations at church you would like to add, if any. One way to do this is to run over in your mind the jobs that will likely have to be done and ask yourself if you feel drawn toward any of them. Another way is to discern which needs call out for your attention by considering them in prayer. To help you determine which needs you should be meeting, you might ask yourself: (1) What is my motivation for committing to this project? Is it guilt, pride, a desire for recognition? Often these emotions are not sufficient to carry you through the course of a project in the spirit of serenity and enthusiasm you desire. (2) If I take on this obligation, will I be so tightly scheduled that I won't have time to rest, relax, or respond spontaneously to some important opportunity that may come up later? We have been impressed by how often those precious moments of fulfillment at Christmas occur in the blank spaces around scheduled events, when you have time to reflect on your experiences and deepen your understanding.

If you are a church leader, you are probably well aware of the oversized load carried by a few people in your congregation at Christmas. Keep this problem in mind when you are thinking of people to fill particular positions. Perhaps your church could make it a practice to seek out good potential leaders and consciously prepare them for responsibility. In many cases, asking people to take on work for the church at Christmas can be a ministry to them. People you know to be lonely or shy or unsure can gain added confidence and much needed social interaction in the process of working for the church. Although many jobs must be done by the most competent person available, others are not so crucial. If you can afford to let the job be done less than perfectly, then ask the people who need to be asked and concentrate your attention on the benefits they are getting, rather than on how the end product looks.

In addition, you may want to consider, with the church community, whether all the activities and events you have scheduled at Christmas really further your ministry or whether they add busyness without adding depth and meaning. The Appendix will give you additional suggestions for effective church programming at Christmas.

When you have considered ahead of time, through prayer and systematic thought, which commitments you are called to take on, you will feel equally confident in saying yes or no when asked. Perhaps the best advice we have read on this subject comes from an essay in the December 1891 *Ladies' Home Journal*:

> It has always seemed to me the most difficult of problems to combine in daily life the two parts of the Christian motto; for the effort to show "goodwill toward men" is only too apt to destroy the "peace," and to make home an uncomfortable place where several over-worked people sleep, eat, and discuss plans. Words written by John Foster early in this century often come to my mind. "If I had the power," he says, "of touching a large part of mankind with a spell, amid all this inane activity, it should be this short sentence, Be Quiet, Be Quiet." Surely home life would be happier and philanthropy more helpful if we would but let the peace of Christ rule in our hearts, and learn that rest is not selfishness, and bustling overwork no true service.

I don't have the time or money to get involved in charity work at Christmas, but I would like my celebration to be less self-serving. What are some simple ways I can help others at Christmas?

Acts of charity don't have to be dramatic departures from your normal routine, or cost money, or take a lot of extra time and effort. One of the simplest and most satisfying ways to benefit others without changing your celebration too much is to buy your gifts from charitable organizations. When you purchase your gifts from church bazaars, third-world craft organizations, local craftsmen, or nonprofit agencies, you are giving a double gift—one to the person who unwraps it on Christmas morning, and one to the charitable organization itself. For a list of national and international charitable organizations that offer Christmas gifts for sale, see pages 184–186.

I don't feel comfortable becoming involved in institutional charities. What are some other simple ways I can reach out to people?

Many people find great satisfaction in initiating acts of kindness within their own circle of family members and friends. Just being especially thoughtful to the people you see all the time can make a difference.

First, ask yourself which person or family that you know would most appreciate some personal contact with you during the season. A walk, a shared meal, a phone call, a letter, some free time while you take over their normal responsibilities, a compliment—all these simple things make the ideal of goodwill come alive at Christmas.

Second, you might ask yourself what nonmaterial gift each member of your family would most appreciate from you this Christmas. Perhaps your spouse would like you to be more relaxed or more involved with him or her; your mother might appreciate it if you were a more attentive listener; your father might welcome it if you paid special attention to one of his interests; and your children would undoubtedly be excited at the prospect of more quiet time alone with you. The possibilities for reaching out to the people around you in quiet, simple ways are endless.

I would like to do something helpful in my own community at Christmas, but I don't know what. How can I get involved?

There are many ways to get directly involved with the needy in your own area at Christmas. The organization that comes immediately to mind is the Salvation Army, which itself is practically a Christmas tradition. For many people, the Christmas season doesn't really begin until they hear the familiar sound of the bell ringer. Although the Salvation Army is active all year long, most of its good works are done during the holidays, when it depends on volunteers and donations to accomplish its goal. During a typical Christmas season, the Salvation Army delivers festive meals to shut-ins and poor people; donates gifts to children; gives Christmas parties in needy neighborhoods; and serves meals to transients, patients in alcoholic-treatment centers, and the families of prisoners.

These special Christmas activities, and the ongoing counseling services it provides in the areas of household budgeting and management and employment possibilities, depend on volunteers. If you want to get involved in any of these activities, call your local Salvation Army office, or write to the national headquarters: The Salvation Army, 799 Bloomfield Avenue, Verona, NJ 07044.

Many other local groups will also be involved in helping people in your community at Christmas. The director of volunteer services at your local hospital will give you information on the ways you can help medical patients. Or you can contact your local police and fire departments, Boy Scout and Girl Scout offices, Lions Club, Volunteers of America, neighborhood church, or United Way office. Many communities also have volunteer bureaus that match those who need help at Christmas with those who can give it.

I have always wanted to visit a nursing home at Christmas, but I don't know how to go about it. Can you help?

First, we should say that not everyone is well suited for nursing home visits. If the thought upsets you, or you feel uncomfortable around older people, there are many other ways to serve. But if you really think you would enjoy such a visit, here are some suggestions to make your visit a success.

✳ Rest assured that one visit is better than none. Even if you can't come regularly, your presence will be appreciated at Christmas.

✳ Let the nursing home staff know you are coming, so they can coordinate visits and prepare the patients. If possible, visit the nursing home on Christmas Eve or Christmas Day, since this is when it is most painful for the patients to be alone.

✳ When you visit, don't be in a hurry. Most patients have time on their hands, and your visit will probably seem too short no matter how long you stay.

✳ Do bring your children. The chance to be around young people is a treat. Children and animals do more to cheer up older people than almost anything else. (You may want to prepare your children for the visit by telling them what to expect.)

✳ If you are lucky enough to have the time and opportunity to develop a continuing relationship with an older person in a nursing home, remember that one of the best gifts you can give is the gift of expectation. Old people often have nothing to look forward to. One woman told us that she had adopted a man in a nursing home and always made it a point to let him know in advance when she would be visiting. That way, he had the pleasure of anticipating her arrival in addition to the pleasure of her company.

✳ After you have developed a friendship with a patient, consider bringing a tape recorder to record his or her life story. One woman told us she did this and typed up the resulting "biography" for her older friend's family.

✳ If you want to bring gifts, remember to provide some for both men and women, wrap each gift and attach a card indicating which sex it is for, and take the gifts to the front desk to ask the receptionist how they should be distributed. Here are some gift ideas:

Live flowers
Useful things such as lap robes, bags for personal belongings, slippers, bibs, pillows, sweaters
Books with large print
An outside excursion to a park or restaurant or the local shops, if the older person is mobile
A deck of cards or other game that you can play together
An offer to mount an older person's family photographs in an album

Do *not* bring candy or cookies without the permission of the nursing home staff. Many older patients are diabetic.

You are riding through the snowy New England countryside in a sleigh pulled by a magnificent team of Clydesdale horses. The only sounds you hear are the footfalls of the horses, the creaking of harnesses, and the ringing of sleigh bells. Your cheeks are red from the rush of cold air, but the wool blankets heaped around you keep you snug and warm. As much as you are enjoying this ride, you are also eager to reach the warm, brightly lit home in the country where you are expected for Christmas dinner. The scenery is so beautiful, and your spirits are so high, that you start humming "I'll Be Home for Christmas" in time to the jingling of the bells.

You finally arrive at your destination, and as you knock on the door of the elegant country house, a television announcer breaks into your reverie. All of a sudden you realize that you are sitting in an armchair watching television, not riding in a horse-drawn sleigh, and that this delightful sixty-second ride through the snow has been brought to you by a certain brand of beer. As the commercial fades away, you are faced once again with the reality of everyday life.

The advertisers who conceived this commercial know what people really want for Christmas. Most people long for a celebration that is just as serene, connected to the natural world, and free of modern distractions as this idyllic sleigh ride through the country. But the fact is, most people are caught up in a labyrinth of holiday plans and projects: There are gifts to buy, packages to mail, cookies to bake, houses to decorate, choir rehearsals to attend, travel plans to make. Many people are so busy that the only time they get out of doors is those few seconds it takes to dash from the house to the car. And their chance for a peaceful celebration is overwhelmed by factors they can't seem to control.

We get a clear picture of how people really want Christmas to be when we ask workshop participants to spend a few minutes fantasizing a perfect holiday. We ask them to imagine what the celebration would be like if they could throw out all their old ideas and habits and start

Chapter
eight

A
SIMPLE
CHRISTMAS

anew with only their personal tastes and preferences to take into account. The only requirement is that they imagine the Christmas that makes them feel most fulfilled.

The fantasies people create turn out to be filled with unique and colorful details. One person will imagine Christmas in the Alps. Another will camp on the beach. Someone else will stay at home but change his everyday environment by unplugging the television and the phone. But the most startling thing about all of the fantasies is that, underneath the eccentric details, most of them are essentially alike. Despite the fact that we urge everyone to give his imagination free rein, nearly everyone comes up with a variation of the same celebration. We have discovered that most people are united by a single Christmas dream. In brief outline, it goes like this:

Snow is falling in a quiet and serene natural setting. Inside the house, a fire glows in the fireplace. There are few modern distractions like televisions, telephones, cars, or radios, and the only holiday decorations are a Christmas tree, candles, greens, and simple homemade decorations. Christmas presents, if there are any, are inexpensive remembrances, or intangible spiritual gifts. The family members are in a good mood and enjoy each other's company in simple ways, like taking walks or sleigh rides together, or gathering around the fire to sing carols or play musical instruments. It doesn't take much to make people laugh, and if there is work to be done, such as the preparation of traditional food, the tasks are shared or completed in some magical way without effort. The children are happy and well behaved and enjoy each other's company. A relaxed, loving atmosphere washes over everyone and awakens them to all the religious or spiritual possibilities that unite them at Christmas.

In this fantasy, there are no elaborate Christmas centerpieces, exotically decorated trees, tables set with Spode Christmas china, or three-hour gift-unwrapping sessions. Most of the activities that require a lot of money and preparation have vanished, so people have the peace of mind to be receptive to each other and the world around them. This universal dream shows that at Christmas people want to be in harmony with the natural world, united with friends and relatives, filled with a spirit of love and acceptance, and have their everyday cares lightened with fun and laughter.

This leads us to an obvious question. If most people are longing for such a simple celebration, why are their holidays so complicated? Why don't more people pare down their activities and obligations until they have the peaceful, spontaneous celebration they envision?

To begin with, there are two factors that stand in the way. First, most people's fantasies involve a little magic. As soon as they close their eyes, they suddenly become the proud owners of a house in the country complete with a fireplace, a sleigh, and a ready team of horses. Or they wake up in the morning blessed with a Christmas snowfall. Fantasies, by their very nature, involve a lot of wishful thinking. And fantasies can't serve as blueprints until they're ruthlessly pruned of all the make-believe.

Second, people cleverly screen out life's unpleasant realities in their fantasies. No one has ever described a fantasy to us in which they had to cope with crying babies, bored teenagers, dirty dishes, or complicated negotiations over who should pay for what. Even the simplest Christmas involves some planning and rearranging of schedules, but no one ever mentions any of these wearisome details. People have an understandable wish to be like children at Christmas, with all of the fun and none of the responsibilities.

But wishful thinking aside, the core of the fantasy—simple gifts, natural decorations, a fire, traditional food, leisurely schedules, music, time spent out of doors, an emphasis on family activities—is well within reach. And we're meeting a lot of people who are moving in this direction. But there are many more who still feel trapped in an expensive, commercial, and complicated Christmas.

Part of the reason more people aren't living out their Christmas dreams is that everywhere they turn they are encouraged to make Christmas as expensive and elaborate and busy as possible. TV commercials show excited children coming downstairs on Christmas morning to a tree heaped with goodies. Magazines urge Mom to make this Christmas one her family will remember by filling the house with lavish decorations. Dads are told to be grateful they have credit cards so they can go into debt to give their families the Christmas they really deserve. The number of days until Christmas is printed in big type on the front pages of newspapers just to make sure everyone is aware of the countdown. The implication is that there's so much to do and buy that everyone must rush to get everything done on time.

Why don't newspapers and magazines and commercials tell people simply to relax and enjoy the holiday? It's not hard to figure out. If everyone decorated with greens, gave token presents to the immediate family only, gathered together for a potluck dinner, and posted a handful of seasonal letters, our national economy would have to make a big adjustment. A simple Christmas is an economic bust.

But it's not just economic pressure that's been keeping Christmas complex. Even while people want to simplify Christmas, they may also have a strong need to keep Christmas the same. Especially when their lives are stressful and subject to change, they want Christmas to be a haven of familiar rituals. And most people today grew up with fairly elaborate celebrations. Even though part of them would like Christmas to be simpler and less commercial, they also want to hold on to the comfort and nostalgia of their childhood Christmases.

Others find that family obligations stand in the way. In their fantasies, most people feel complete freedom to pick and choose from the family roster the group of relatives they want to spend Christmas with. And, of course, in their daydreams, everyone on this handpicked list goes along with their plans. In real life, it's not that simple. For example, a woman named Hillary told us that her husband's parents were ailing and counted on her a great deal to help them out at Christmas. She and her husband spent many days helping clean and decorate their house, going shopping for them, and cheering them up.

Hillary told us that this was not the way she would choose to spend Christmas if she had only her own wishes to consider. When she imagined a perfect holiday, she saw her family going to the beach or to a mountain cabin. They were all outdoors people and longed to be away from the city and free from the demands of others. Nevertheless, it was more important to her to be accommodating. "My in-laws have no other family," she told us. "We're all they have. And family is what Christmas is all about. I'm glad to do it for them."

But Hillary, like most people, was able to hold on to the spirit of her fantasy Christmas despite her family obligations. She told us that on Christmas Day she was able to leave the grandparents with a cousin and take a long walk in the park with her husband and children. "The park was quiet and empty," she told us, "and we felt as peaceful as if we were in the middle of the woods."

We've met a lot of people, however, who are able to live out their entire holiday fantasies.

This was the case for a sixty-five-year-old woman named Katharine who masterminded a plan to gather three generations of her family together for a simple Christmas celebration at the beach. She saw the need for change when she looked around her one Christmas and saw that most of the family was just going through the motions of having a good time. "Especially the teenagers," she said. "They were pretty obviously bored with the whole thing." She spent some time after Christmas thinking about what would make her family most happy and decided it was a simple Christmas on the Oregon coast. In the summer, Katharine proposed to the family that they combine their Christmas money and rent a cabin at the beach for the coming holiday. She suggested that they not exchange gifts and simplify the cooking by bringing along precooked potluck dishes. Everyone in the family was excited by the idea, and someone even suggested that they bring along materials to make ornaments for a tree.

Despite the fact that Katharine was the one who came up with the idea of not exchanging gifts, she told us that she got two beautiful Christmas presents all the same. One was the fact that a grandson took her for a walk on the beach to tell her it was the best Christmas of his life. And the other was waking up on Christmas morning, looking out the window, and seeing that her grandchildren had written MERRY CHRISTMAS GRANDMA in ten-foot letters in the sand.

Katharine and her family discovered that even dramatically simplifying their celebration did not take away any of its value. In fact, they all agreed it was the best Christmas they had ever spent together. No one was burdened with long hours in the kitchen. All of them had time to relax and talk in depth with each other. And while they had been worried at first about how Christmas would feel without gifts, they felt relieved to be free from all the worry and expense of gift giving.

Whether you live out your Christmas dream in every detail or find one small part to incorporate, taking the time to create the fantasy is one of the most important steps you can take. Your fantasies can give you a new enthusiasm for Christmas and the sense of direction you need to start building a better celebration.

In the following exercise, you will have a chance to visualize the kind of Christmas *you* really want. Then we will answer typical questions people have when they're thinking about simplifying their celebrations. In addition, the Appendix offers specific suggestions for simplifying your decorations, Christmas cards, entertaining, gift giving, and food preparation.

Exercise

A CHRISTMAS FANTASY

The following fantasy exercise will give you a clearer idea of what you are really looking for in Christmas. When you are through reading these instructions, close your eyes and imagine Christmas two years from now. We have chosen this length of time because it's far enough away to give you some distance from your current celebration, but not so far away that a lot of your circumstances will have changed.

When you are ready to begin, choose a quiet location where you won't be interrupted for ten or fifteen minutes. Imagine any kind of Christmas you wish as long as it is deeply satisfying. You can confine your fantasy to Christmas proper, or include the whole season. It may be very much like your present celebration or entirely different. You can magically include your favorite friends and relatives and make them behave any way you wish. You can celebrate in any setting. You don't have to keep a single traditional Christmas activity, or you can keep them all. This will be Christmas the way you have always wanted it to be.

As you begin to fantasize, there will probably be a jumble of possibilities competing for your attention. If you find yourself with multiple fantasies, keep returning to the ideas that make you feel most satisfied.

Once you have settled on a particular fantasy, stick with it until you have enriched it with lots of details. Imagine the physical setting, the activities, how you are feeling, and how other people are feeling. What kind of food is there? How was it made? Are there any gifts? What are they like?

When you have completed your fantasy, write it down on a separate sheet (or sheets) of paper. Feel free to elaborate as you write. Then answer these questions:

1 Of all the ways your fantasy was different from your usual celebration, which difference was most satisfying to you?

2 Which parts (if any) of your fantasy would be most feasible to actually do next Christmas?

People often get a great deal of pleasure from reading the fantasies of others. Here is a sampling from those we have collected:

A few days before Christmas, Grace and the kids and I pack *leisurely* and go up to a mountain cabin. The roads are packed with snow but surprisingly drivable. The kids don't know where we're going, but Grace does, and she's *relaxed*. We talk. We talk about some things past and some things future. Then we arrive at a comfortable, real log cabin in a pine forest.

The kids are excited but well behaved. We unload and settle in in no time flat. There are no hassles getting the kids fed or getting them to take a nap. We are all relaxed.

The next few days pass in wonderful, calm togetherness. Romps in the snow. Wonderful but not overstuffed meals. Then on Christmas Eve we all bundle up and go to a nearby town for a midnight Christmas service. The kids fall asleep in our arms and are perfect angels. The service is calm, peaceful, hopeful, and full of Christmas music.

In the morning Ben and Margaret drive up to spend the day. Both sets of kids are overjoyed to see each other but are still well behaved. My mother in-law arrives later in the day. Football on TV. A turkey in the oven. Rest. Joy. Fellowship.

For my perfect Christmas we would go and live in a log cabin at the beginning of December. It would be snowing and we would travel by sleigh. We would cut down our own tree and have no electricity. For Christmas my mom and dad would get me my own horse and I would go off riding by myself in the snow.

The days would be cold and clear and the snow would not melt for a long time. We would make our own ornaments and have hardwood floors. We would have wheat, corn, eggs, and other things and we would live there until school started again.

My perfect Christmas would happen by accident. Nobody would even know it was Christmas. All my family would happen to converge on a big house in a good mood with a few days to spend together.

It would be nobody's house, so no one person would feel

responsible for cleaning and decorating it or fixing it up for company. We'd all go for a walk in the woods and bring evergreen boughs and holly back to the house because we liked the smells. And because there's no electricity, the house would glow with candlelight.

Someone would have brought a special bottle of red wine, and we'd sit down to a simple but wonderful meal. We'd be in such a relaxed and open mood, and would have had such a good day walking in the woods, that someone would propose a toast and say, "This is such a fine day, it feels just like Christmas." Then we'd all smile and clink our glasses together, feeling warm and together.

There would be no talk of Jesus, but we would be very loving and accepting of ourselves and each other. For the first time we would have the sensation of seeing each other at our best.

In the morning, we'd wake up to a snowy day. No one had expected this snowfall, and even the weather report hadn't predicted it. It was a gift. And as we sat around having a late and relaxed breakfast, someone would rush to his suitcase with something he had brought for another person—not a wrapped present, just something he thought the other person would enjoy: a special book, a drawing, a new recipe. . . . There would be something for everyone.

A day later, we'd all take a final, exhilarating walk in the snowy woods. And then all would pack up and go home, never knowing that it was Christmas, but feeling happy and at peace.

When people in our workshops describe their visions of a perfect Christmas, we usually hear wonderfully detailed fantasies—a ski trip in the Rockies, a country Christmas in Vermont, or delightful variations on specific family rituals. But one woman was able to capture her dream for a better Christmas in just a few words. "I have only one request," she said, "and that's for Christmas to bring my family closer together. I want us to have fun together, not sit in separate corners of the room reading magazines or watching TV." As she said this, she stretched her arms out to her sides and then slowly brought them together in a big circle, as if to gather up her scattered family.

As she explained her wish, she told us that every Christmas her family went through the same sterile routine. "On Christmas Eve, I'm in the kitchen cooking while everyone else is reading magazines or watching TV. Then we eat. Then a few people help me clean up and it's back to the television. The next morning, we open the gifts. Then I cook breakfast. The dishes are cleaned up. And then it's more TV and sports magazines. Then I'm back in the kitchen again, cooking dinner."

This bleak portrayal of a family Christmas is all too familiar to us. Many of the people that we've talked to spend their holiday opening gifts, sitting, talking, eating, drinking, listening to other people sing, watching other people play ball games on TV, and watching television specials. At times, it seems as if we, as a nation, have lost the art of celebrating.

Our passive American way of Christmas seems even more flat and empty when we compare it to the lively folk festivals of other countries. For example, in one workshop, a man named José who had recently emigrated from Mexico volunteered to tell us about his childhood Christmas. Most of his memories centered on Los Posados, the Mexican Christmas festival that reenacts Joseph and Mary's search for an inn and lasts from December 16 until Christmas Day. José explained that on each of the nine nights of the celebration, a different family invited the villagers in for an evening of singing, treats, and a chance to break a piñata.

José had especially fond memories of the last night of the festival, when his female relatives gathered in one kitchen to make tamales and traditional Mexican sweets. As soon as the food was ready, the whole neighborhood got together and partied until daybreak. "There was dancing and drinks for the adults and hot punch and games for the kids," he said. When he was through, we asked how the American Christmas seemed to him, and José answered that it looked pretty sad. Every holiday he wished he could fly his family back to Mexico. "In Mexico, we had Christmas," he said. "In the United States, you just have presents."

Our modern version of Christmas seems just as uninspired when compared to celebrations of the past. In Victorian England, for example, families celebrated Christmas with an exuberant collection of games— blindman's buff, charades, snapdragon, and hunt the slipper—where *all* family members took part, not just the children. You can sense their joy in the following excerpts from *The Victorian Christmas Book* by Anthony and Peter Miall (New York: Pantheon Books, 1978): "A speckled physician of sixty sitting on his hams on a carpet, and passing the slipper under him, with all the dexterity, if not with all the glee, of a school boy, is a sight to be enjoyed."

After the games and elaborate, full-costume charades, there were conjuring tricks, recitations, and singing. And then came the dancing: "Hark! the sound of music: the Christmas dance begins; and Polka— the universal polka—summons all hands and feet to another celebration; and to a sport in comparison to which all others are of small account."

The vitality of the English family Christmas was equaled by the celebrations of early Americans. A hundred years ago, our great grand-parents spent their Christmas vacations sleighing, skating, caroling, and masquerading, and when they came inside with red cheeks and high spirits, they played parlor games or rolled back the carpets and invited the neighbors over for a dance.

Learning about the traditions, games, and activities that delighted our ancestors provides clues to the current widespread nostalgia for an old fashioned Christmas. It's not just the trappings of yesterday's celebrations that people want—prairie dresses for their little girls, Colonial ornaments for their trees, authentic reproductions of sleigh bells for their front doors—it's the very life and spirit of past celebrations that they hunger for. The consumer's, spectator's celebration of today is dreary by comparison. For many of the people we talk to, Christmas is often just a little bit more of the things they are used to all year round—more food, more people, more material goods. But nothing dramatically different. The folk traditions and family activities that added so much mystery and cadence to the holiday have been largely forgotten.

What has happened to them all? As recently as the middle of the nineteenth century, they were intact. All around the country there were pockets of Spanish, German, English, French, Scandinavian, and Dutch Christmas celebrations. In fact, until the late 1800s there was no such thing as a distinct American Christmas. But by the turn of the century, the population had become more integrated, and the various national customs began to merge together.

Because of this amalgamation, a modern family celebration may contain traces of five or six different cultures. A family may decorate the tree with gingerbread cookies like the Germans, have oyster stew on Christmas Eve like the French, have a piñata party for the children like the Mexicans, and eat plum pudding for Christmas dinner like the English. There is no doubt that this bountiful inheritance adds vitality to the American Christmas, because it gives people so many wonderful traditions to pick and choose from. But in some ways, the absence of a single body of traditions makes things more difficult, because each family must assume full responsibility for piecing together a coherent celebration. In addition, because each family makes slightly different choices, there's no chance for the communitywide celebrations that bring such joy in countries like Mexico. Ultimately, each family must rely on its own energy and imagination to define its traditions and keep them alive.

With such diluted traditions, and so little reinforcement for preserving them, it's no wonder that the common denominator of American Christmas celebrations is holiday commercialism. In fact, it could be said that our national celebration begins with the opening ritual of going Christmas shopping the day after Thanksgiving and closes with the hallowed tradition of returning unwanted gifts on December 26. And in between, our citywide observances of Christmas are confined to come-hither "holiday events" in shopping malls.

Families without strong family or ethnic traditions often rely on Christmas commercialism to provide the structure and meaning of their celebrations, depending on an elaborate gift exchange and the passive consumption of media events for the bulk of their fun and excitement. This was the story of a twenty-five-year-old woman named Melissa. For years, the members of her family had focused most of their energy on buying presents for each other, but like many other people, they didn't find this entirely satisfying. "We were sick of all the commercialism," Melissa told us. "Gifts made sense when we were kids, but we were now all adults, so we wanted to do away with some of the trappings." In the fall of 1980, she and her boyfriend, her parents, and her older brother decided to celebrate Christmas by just getting together for a visit and a smorgasbord brunch.

But when Melissa and her family took away the gifts and the elaborate decorations, they found they had little left. "We had a beautiful meal," Melissa said, "and then went out to the living room to talk. It was pleasant. But we all had the feeling that there was something missing." While they enjoyed each other's company and were relieved not to be overburdened with all the details of gift giving, the celebration seemed empty. As Melissa told us, "Christmas is an existential abyss."

Many people are eager to eliminate some of the more commercial aspects of their family celebrations, but like Melissa's family, they don't want to end up with a bare-bones Christmas either. They want a vital and fun-filled celebration that fully measures up to all those weeks of anticipation. They want to let go of parts of Christmas that have little meaning to them, but they also want to find some way to live out the joy and excitement of the holiday season.

What can families do to add to the merriment of their celebrations? By looking to the past, exploring other cultures, and talking with people in this country who have wonderful Christmases, we have learned that there are some simple, inexpensive, and noncommercial ways to enliven the holiday.

One of the first is to make sure that every family member has a vital role to play in the traditions the family already has. People generally take the most pleasure in activities they are really involved in. But all too often, as we pointed out in the earlier chapters, women play most of the key roles in the family production while the other family members are passive recipients of all of their labors.

A Portland, Oregon, family found a way to get everyone more involved in the celebration. One year, three adult sisters were discussing their Christmas reunion plans when one of them suggested that they eliminate the traditional Christmas brunch. In the past, when all three families congregated, it had meant cooking up a meal for eighteen people, and that was a lot of extra work for the women. One of the husbands overheard this proposal and made a mild protest. It just wouldn't be Christmas, he said, without that traditional meal. His wife quickly suggested that the men make the brunch that year. The three husbands got together for a quick consultation and decided to accept the challenge.

That Christmas, when all the gifts had been unwrapped, the three men trooped into the kitchen, closed the door behind them, and started cooking. The women were grateful to have a chance to sit in the living room, play with the children, and admire the presents. Two hours later, the men called everyone into the dining room and presented the family with a beautiful brunch that featured grilled trout and pancakes. The meal was superb and the men's pride was obvious.

The following year, the men decided to make this an annual event. And they got the children involved by asking them to be responsible for setting the table. On their own, the children decided to make a centerpiece, a handprinted menu, and place cards. By giving the men and children more active roles in the celebration, this family created a fun-filled tradition.

A second step families can take to recapture the spirit of Christmas is to include activities that add movement and physical activity to the celebration. As we've read accounts of past Christmases, we've been struck by how often the holiday was observed with enthusiastic bursts of energy. Whether it was through dancing, mime, parading, or putting on plays, people broke stride with the daily round of work and rest by participating in high-spirited activities that got them all up and moving.

Today, you can find this kind of physical activity in any number of ways. You can walk to the store to get that extra pound of butter, or play charades instead of sitting around watching TV. Or you can do something as ambitious as renting a ski lodge in the mountains over Christmas vacation. We recently heard about a large extended family that pools its resources and rents a ski lodge in the Colorado mountains every year. Each of the separate families gladly simplifies its gift giving in order to save money for the annual stay at the lodge.

A skiing Christmas works for this group on a number of different levels. Each family unit can come and go whenever it wants, there is no pressure to exchange gifts, and, best of all, there is ample opportunity for each of the thirty or so people who gather at the lodge to enjoy some physical activity. Most of the adults spend the better part of each day cross-country skiing, while less physically active people stay behind to supervise the younger children's play in the snow. One way or another, everyone gets a much appreciated breath of fresh air.

This is such an important tradition for this family that the two grandmothers have both willed portions of their estates to provide future funds for renting the lodge.

A third thing families can do is look for lighthearted ways to add fun to their celebrations. Solemn moments have their place at Christmas, but there are also many opportunities for laughter, even silliness. For example, one family has started the tradition of passing around, year after year, the same grotesque tie. Each year, the person who received the tie the year before wraps it up and presents it to some other member of the family. The trick is to disguise it so well that no one can guess which package it's in. One year, the tie was baked in a cake; another year it was worked into the design of a wall hanging.

Finally, some people find that they can add more excitement and meaning to their holiday rituals by reaching back into the past and reviving traditions from their ethnic heritage. One woman, whose ancestors were from England, became so intrigued with the idea of a real mince pie that she learned how to make one using beef and suet. "I always used to serve mince pie," she told us, "but I would just reach for a jar on my shelf, twist off the lid, and fill a packaged pie shell. I never realized the care that went into making a real one. All the time I was chopping the meat, I was thinking that my grandmother probably did this every year for Christmas. I felt very close to her."

Sometimes finding ways to be more genuinely excited about Christmas takes some extra thought and effort. But when people value what they are doing, the added "work" becomes part of the fun of Christmas.

Of the two exercises in this chapter, we want to draw your attention especially to Making a Plan on page 132. This exercise will help you incorporate all the insights you've gained from reading this book into a simple plan for a more satisfying, joyful Christmas. We urge you to take the time to complete this particular exercise so you will have a clear sense of direction during the coming holiday season. This planning process is an essential component of our group workshops and one that we highly recommend to readers of this book.

Following the exercises, you will find many pages of suggestions for simple games, traditions, and activities to add more life to your celebration. Most of these cost little or no money and require very little preparation time. Whether your family is large or small, intellectual or athletic, reserved or riotous, we hope you will find at least one or two ways to have a merrier Christmas.

Exercises

FAMILY FUN

This exercise will help you clarify what kinds of activities your family most enjoys and will give you some ideas for new traditions to liven up your holiday.

1 Which of the following activities are generally enjoyed by the people you celebrate Christmas with? Check those you participated in last Christmas.

- ✳ Doing winter sports (specify)
- ✳ Card playing
- ✳ Game playing
- ✳ Singing
- ✳ Playing musical instruments
- ✳ Reading aloud to each other
- ✳ Attending concerts
- ✳ Entertaining friends
- ✳ Telling anecdotes about the family
- ✳ Dancing
- ✳ Cooking together
- ✳ Going for walks
- ✳ Taking trips to the country
- ✳ Creating skits and plays
- ✳ Caroling

2 Star the activities that you would like to do this year.

By doing this exercise, many people realize that they often neglect many of their favorite activities at Christmas. Adding just one enjoyable tradition is often all it takes to have a more rewarding celebration.

MAKING A PLAN

There are several ideas to keep in mind as you go about creating a plan for the coming Christmas celebration. First, as you make your plan, you should realize that this blueprint will not be your only instrument of change. You will probably find yourself making numerous small adjustments in your celebration that are too insignificant to mention in your plan. All of these moment-by-moment decisions will add up to a more enjoyable celebration. Your plan is merely a tool to help you focus on the important changes you wish to make.

Second, set small and specific goals. Our experience has shown us that people need time to adjust to new ideas—especially in an area of their lives where traditions play such an important role. Therefore, modest plans tend to be most successful. Besides, many people find that they don't want to change all that much about the way they celebrate Christmas. They just want to clear away a few activities that have lost meaning, add a tradition or two, and look for more depth and spirit in their established rituals.

Third, the time of year when you are making this plan is going to play a key role in determining your goals. If you are planning in midsummer, you have the time to make changes that involve a lot of people, such as talking to all family members about giving fewer or simpler gifts. If you are making your plan a week before Christmas, you need to set your sights on changes that can be enacted at the last minute, such as adding a new family activity the day after Christmas that will help your children gradually wind down from all the excitement.

Fourth, you will have greater success if you focus on goals that you can accomplish independently, or that have the likely support of everyone involved. For example, if you are bothered by a relative's excessive drinking, you will probably be frustrated if you define your goal this way: "I would like to encourage my father to drink less this Christmas." A more realistic goal statement would be: "I would like to add activities to our celebration that would take the emphasis off drinking." This second goal is one that you could accomplish even without your father's cooperation.

The first step in actually making your written Christmas plan is to bring to mind your most important ideas for change. Take out a sheet of paper and list those ideas.

Next, select two or three of the most important and realistic ideas to incorporate this season. How do you make this choice? We have found that the fantasy exercise on page 122 often gives people the best indication of what's most important to them about Christmas. You may also find it helpful to ask yourself these questions:

1 If my goals involve other family members, am I likely to have their support?

2 Do I have the time and resources to accomplish these goals this year?

3 Will fulfilling these goals keep intact all the parts of my celebration that have strong emotional appeal to me and others?

If you answered yes to all three of these questions, chances are you have realistic goals. If you found some difficulties, stop to revise your goals before going on to the next step.

For some examples of good goal sentences, look through this list that we collected at the end of one of our workshops:

∗ I want to minimize Christmas preparations.

∗ I want to feel more relaxed this holiday season.

∗ I want to simplify my gift giving.

∗ I want to spend more relaxed time with my children this Christmas.

∗ I want to give less commercial gifts.

When you have two or three workable goals, your next step is to decide exactly how you're going to reach them. So far, you may only have a general idea of what you're aiming for. Look at your goals and think of one, two, or three activities that will help you accomplish them. Remember that unless you are assured of other people's cooperation, it's best to focus on activities that you can do by yourself.

Next you need to describe these activities in simple written sentences. These sentences should tell you exactly *what* you are going to do and *when* it should be done. Here is an example:

Goal: I want to simplify my gift giving.

Activity 1: I will write letters to Aunt Carol and Aunt Rebecca suggesting that we give gifts only to the children and mail those letters by October 1.

Activity 2: I will talk with my friends at work this week and suggest that we go out to lunch together instead of exchanging Christmas presents.

Activity 3: I will do all of my gift shopping for the children from the Childcraft catalogue and phone in the order by the end of October.

When you have finished choosing activities for all of your goals and checked to make sure they are small and specific, have family support, and are fixed in a specific time frame, you are through. You may want to keep your plan tacked up on the refrigerator or on the bulletin board, where you will be reminded of it and you can cross off each activity as it's completed.

Now that you have your plan, how do you share it with your family?

You, of course, are the best judge of how to approach them. You may have relatives who are likely to be supportive of all your ideas and will require only a quick phone call to fill them in on the details. On the other hand, you may have family members who will need to hear your reasons for seeking change and then have time to think about it. Only you know which is the case.

But we do have some general recommendations for talking to family members about making changes. First, choose your time carefully. Wait until people are in a relaxed and accepting frame of mind before you launch into your ideas. Second, be nonthreatening. Unless the other family members have done a lot of thinking about Christmas, introduce the topic gently. Third, take the time to explain your reasons for wanting to make changes. Once people know the sincere motivations behind your plan, they are likely to be more supportive. And finally, talk to others as soon as possible. Many people like to plan for Christmas early.

Questions and Answers

Even though my family is all together in one physical location at Christmas, we seem to stay emotionally distant. Is there any way to bring us all together?

Some families are naturally outgoing, but others need a little encouragement. First, to set the stage, check to make sure that your family celebration has neither too many activities nor too few. When there's too much going on, people often have to retreat inside themselves to find peace of mind. And when there are too few activities, people tend to become bored and seek refuge in solitary pursuits.

Second, you may want to add a family ritual through which you can express your love in a more direct way than giving gifts. In many countries, people have Christmas traditions that help them openly show their affection. In Poland, for example, families share special crackers (Oplateks) embossed with the Nativity scene before Christmas Eve dinner. When the ceremony begins, each family member is given a wafer. Then the father and mother embrace and express their love for each other, and each takes a bite from the other's Oplatek. This ritual is repeated until each person has shared his Oplatek and a few kind words with every other family member. Sharing of the Oplatek is so important to Poles that they mail crackers to relatives and close friends who are unable to join them at Christmas.

Consider beginning *your* Christmas dinner with a special ritual to remind you of why you are all together. It can be as simple as a prayer, a toast, a candle-lighting ceremony, or just a few quiet moments holding hands.

In addition, here are some more ideas to bring your family closer together: Ask family members to bring items for a "Family Museum." Suitable things would be old photographs, diaries, heirlooms, written anecdotes, or genealogical information. Display them in a central place and people will be brought together to talk about family history.

After dinner, tell family anecdotes. Who can tell the earliest one? Who has a story no one has ever heard before? How many versions are there of the same family story? (You may want to tape this session.)

If you have home movies or videotapes of your family, bring them out and play them for the assembled relatives. Everyone likes to see how people have grown and changed.

How can we add more excitement to our holiday food? It's not very inspired.

You may find that simply adding more drama and ceremony to your traditional food will make it more fun for everyone. In the past, there were elaborate rituals surrounding the preparation and presentation of many holiday foods. For example, here is an account of how eggnog was made on a Southern plantation, according to a December 1889 *Ladies' Home Journal*:

> By the time our stockings were emptied and examined, grandpa, fully dressed, had come out of his room into the hall where . . . all the material for making eggnog had been set out on a gigantic scale—a fanner of fresh eggs, great dishes of sugar, and the cellaret of liquors. When the eggs were beaten to the required degree, viz., until the yolks were the color of rich cream and the whites adhered steadily to the dish when it was turned upside down, the whole was put together in the gigantic china punch-bowl, relic of ancestral feastings across seas in "ye old Countrie." I would not dare to say how many eggs, or how much brandy and rum went into the concoction of that bowl of eggnog. When it was pronounced right, a waiter of glasses was filled and handed round to the assembled company; and then "the stand" —a great circular, claw-footed mahogany table—was lifted out on the wide front piazza, the flaming sconces were lighted, and the eggnog bowl, surrounded by pyramids of tumblers, was placed upon it. Then we proceeded to "drink in Christmas."

Our modern way of serving eggnog is to buy it ready-made in cartons at the grocer's and serve it anytime from Thanksgiving to New Year's. If you like eggnog, consider making it from scratch on Christmas Day. You will probably find yourself serving your homemade nog with more pride and ceremony.

Be on the lookout for ways to add drama to your other holiday favorites, too. For example, if you traditionally serve plum pudding at Christmas, douse it with warm brandy, light it, turn down the dining room lights, and bring the pudding in with proper pomp and circumstance. For added interest, you may want to use this adaptation of an authentic recipe, which was judged the best of five hundred entries submitted to a London newspaper in 1876:

PROPER PLUM PUDDING

MAKES 6 POUNDS

✳ ——————————————

1 pound currants
1 pound raisins
1 pound suet (modern tastes might prefer less suet)
¾ pound dried bread crumbs
½ a nutmeg, grated (about 1 teaspoon)
¼ pound brown sugar

1 *lemon rind, grated*
½ *pound minced, candied orange peel*
5 *eggs*
½ *pint brandy*

Clean, wash, and dry the currants and raisins. Mix the suet and all the dry ingredients together. Beat the eggs, add them to the brandy, then pour over the dry ingredients and mix thoroughly. Pack into small greased kettles or molds and steam for 6 hours. Serve with hard sauce or brandy sauce.

A final way to make your holiday food more enjoyable is to involve more people in its preparation. Set aside a leisurely afternoon, gather several friends or family members, put a Christmas record on the turntable, and make one of your favorite recipes. You may want to reenact a pioneer Christmas tradition and invite a dozen friends in for a taffy pull. There are few cooking activities that can happily involve so many people. One person can mix the ingredients. Another can monitor the candy thermometer. Two people can cut the paper to wrap the candies. Young children can butter the cooking trays. Everyone will want turns pulling the taffy. And when the taffy is done, all hands can sit around a table to shape and wrap the candy. Here is a recipe for vanilla taffy and five ways to change the flavoring.

✳ ─────────────────────

TAFFY

MAKES 2 POUNDS

1 *ounce unsweetened chocolate (optional)*
2½ *cups sugar*
1½ *cups light corn syrup*
1⅓ *cups water*
2 *tablespoons vinegar*
1 *teaspoon salt*
¼ *cup butter, plus more to butter the pans*
2 *teaspoons vanilla (omit for some of the variations)*
  Cornstarch

Have someone butter two baking pans with rims to receive the hot taffy syrup. (If you want to make chocolate taffy, grate 1 ounce of unsweetened chocolate over the bottom of the tray.) Combine all the ingredients except the butter and flavoring in a heavy 3-quart saucepan. Cook and stir over low heat until the sugar is dissolved. Turn the burner on high and cook without stirring until the candy reaches 265°F. Remove from the heat and add the butter. Pour carefully into the buttered pans. (Make sure children are far away from the very hot syrup.)

Cool until a dent remains when you press your finger into the syrup. Sprinkle on the flavoring, butter your hands or coat them with cornstarch, and gather the taffy into your hands. (Make sure it is cool enough to handle.) Pull it into long ropes, double over, and pull again, until the taffy loses some of its gloss, turns lighter in color, and becomes stiffer, and ridges appear on the ropes as you stretch it out. Cut the long taffy ropes into small pieces with buttered scissors. Shape into cubes, balls, or ovals and wrap individually in waxed paper or plastic wrap. (You will want lots of help with the shaping and wrapping, for otherwise it becomes tedious.)

Variations: Add grated chocolate; keep the vanilla. Add grated chocolate and 2 teaspoons of instant coffee; keep the vanilla. Add 1½ cups chopped nuts; keep the vanilla. Omit the vanilla; add ½ teaspoon peppermint extract. Omit the vanilla; add ¼ teaspoon cinnamon oil and red food coloring.

If making taffy seems too ambitious, how about roasting some chestnuts on an open fire (or in your oven if you don't have a fireplace)? To roast chestnuts, cut a cross in the flat side of the chestnut and place near (not in) the coals of an open fire until done. Stir them around once or twice to even out the heat. Or place on a cookie sheet in a 350°F oven for 20 minutes. Take off the shells, salt, and eat as a snack, or dip in chocolate for dessert.

Finally, if you usually go to church on Christmas Eve, have a special midnight supper when you come home (called a *Réveillon* in France). A traditional French menu might include cassoulet (a poultry and bean casserole that can bake in the oven while you are at church), fresh French bread, cheese, a nice bottle of wine or champagne, and *bûche de Noël* (a Yule log cake that is sponge cake filled with buttercream and decorated with chocolate buttercream). You will find recipes for cassoulet and *bûche de Noël* in most comprehensive American cookbooks. Or make it simple. Have omelets, French bread, and cheese.

What are some good games to play at Christmas?

Each family has its own style of game playing. Some like deadly serious games of bridge or backgammon, while others like noisy poker games or board games such as Clue or Pictionary. But since we've observed that family Christmases could stand a good dose of levity, here are two especially silly, unserious games for you to consider. These simple card games can be played by all family members six or older.

"Spoons" is usually regarded as a children's game, but if adults can be encouraged to abandon their reserve, everyone should have a rousing time. To play, you will need a deck of cards and some teaspoons—one fewer than you have players. Before you begin, sort the cards into piles of like numbers. You will use as many sets of four as you have players. Set aside the remaining cards.

Deal out the cards around the circle until each player has four cards, and place the spoons in the middle of the table so that each player has quick access to a spoon. The object of the game is to get all four cards of the same number. When the game begins, the players look at their cards, choose one card each to discard, and pass the discards simultaneously to the players on their left. The players examine their new cards, choose their discards, and then on cue pass them to the left again. The first person to get four of a kind grabs (or sneaks) a spoon. As soon as one spoon is taken, anyone can grab, and the person who isn't quick enough to get one is retired from the game. (You can give the youngest children a handicap by placing spoons especially close to them.)

At the end of each hand, one player, one spoon, and one set of cards is removed from the game, until the last hand, when only two players, one spoon, and two sets of four remain. The winner is the first one to get four of a kind and grab the last spoon.

"I doubt it," another game you may remember from your childhood, gains an added dimension when played by a mixture of children and conniving adults. For this game, you will need a deck of cards and three or four players, or two decks of cards and five to eight players, or three decks of cards and eight to twelve players.

Deal out all the cards. The first person to the left of the dealer begins by taking from one to four cards (one to eight if you are using two decks and one to twelve if you are using three decks) from his hand and placing them facedown in the middle of the table, declaring, "Aces." The second player takes from one to four cards from his hand and places them facedown in the middle of the table, saying, "Twos." The third player does the same, declaring, "Threes." Each player must play at least one card, continuing the sequence of numbers.

The object of the game is to get rid of your cards while declaring them to be the next number in sequence. Since you do not have to reveal the true identity of the cards as you lay them down, you can be either telling the truth or bluffing.

But if someone suspects that you are bluffing, he can say, "I doubt it." Then you have to turn over the cards you just put down and show their true value. If you were telling the truth and all the cards are the number you declared them to be, the person who doubted you has to put into his hand all the cards in the middle of the table. If you were bluffing, however, *you* have to pick up all the cards. The first person to lay down all his cards wins.

There are plenty of other good games. If you have very young children at your celebration, play this variation of hide the thimble. While a child is out of the room, hide a small candy cane. When he returns, everyone should sing "Jingle Bells" loudly (when he's getting warm) or softly (when he's cold) to lead him to the candy cane.

Then, when the children are tucked away in bed, play a game that was a great Victorian Christmas favorite: snapdragon. Here is how the game was described in the *Illustrated London News* a hundred years ago:

> The large pewter dish filled with spirit [brandy] is placed on the floor and attracts the attention of all the party. The light is applied—the flame burns beautifully azure, tipped with amber and scarlet, and whisks and frisks in a manner delightful to contemplate. . . . Throw in the plums [currants]. The spirit burns, the dish is a lake of fire; and he who can gather the prize from the jaws of perils is welcome to it. "Fortune favours the bold!" "Faint heart never won a plum!"

The object is to pluck a glowing currant and pop it into your mouth before your fingers are burned by the "snapdragon."

If your family likes to play charades, organize an elaborate charade party for the day after Christmas. In Victorian England, the charade parties on Boxing Day (December 26) were often looked forward to as much as Christmas itself.

If you're not up to charades, buy your family a new board game or a jigsaw puzzle to be opened on December 26. Then you can draw the family together and have a good way to wind down from the festivities.

I'd like to read aloud to my family at Christmastime. What are some good reading selections?

Before the days of television, reading aloud was a favorite family pastime. Christmas is a good time to revive this custom. You might want to start with a simple Christmas story you won't find anywhere else. We discovered this pioneer letter at the Oregon Historical Society. It was written by a man named George Hines.

> I am reminded of my first Christmas in Oregon, in 1853. My parents and the four of us children had just arrived in Oregon in October of that year. We had no money and only the clothes we had worn across the plains. We were loaned an old cabin to live in until we could build our own, and Father and I dug potatoes on shares for the man who owned the cabin.
>
> All that winter we ate potatoes and boiled wheat and drank rain water.
>
> In December, my sister and I began thinking about Christmas. I thought the prospect was pretty poor, and when we spoke to my mother, she gave us little encouragement. Dad was away working and we barely had enough to eat. All our shoes had holes.
>
> But on Christmas Eve, Mother told us to hang up our stockings. I had no socks, but Mother made a kind of pocket to serve the purpose out of a coat, the sleeves of which I had worn to shreds. So my sister's stockings, very much darned, and my pocket were hung on pegs behind the stove, and we crept into our trundle beds.
>
> Christmas morning came, and I built a fire in the old stove, and by the light of the pitch sticks, I discovered that there was something in our stockings. She found a doughnut doll baby, and an apple. I had an ordinary doughnut and an apple in mine.
>
> It is doubtful that there will ever be more joy in the hearts of any children on Christmas morning.

You can also go to the library and check out one of these classics: *A Child's Christmas in Wales* by Dylan Thomas; *Old Christmas* by Washington Irving; "A Christmas Carol" by Charles Dickens; "The Gift of the Magi" by O. Henry; *A Christmas Memory* by Truman Capote. For children: *On the Banks of Plum Creek* by Laura Ingalls Wilder; *Little Women* by Louisa May Alcott; "The Fir Tree" by Hans Christian Andersen; *Amahl and the Night Visitors* by Gian-Carlo Menotti; "A Visit from St. Nicholas" by Clement Moore.

Our family celebration seems like a blur of people and activities. How can we slow down enough to enjoy Christmas and each other?

One of the best ways to focus the group's energy is to vary the pace of the day. Try alternating physical action with more subdued activities like reading together or telling family anecdotes.

The family gift opening can be either a frenzy of torn paper or a centered, delightful experience. If yours is a Christian family, consider beginning your present opening by reading the Christmas story in Luke. Then open the presents one at a time and take time to appreciate each one. Show young people photographs of faraway relatives who sent them gifts and say a little about them.

Finally, even if you don't normally go to church, you may find that attending a Christmas service will add peace and harmony to your family celebration.

I enjoy Christmas music, but all we do is listen to it. How can I get my family more interested in singing?

Although they may not always admit it, most people like to sing. Often all it takes is one brave soul to get things going. Gather around the piano or sing your favorite carols a cappella. Add to the general merriment by trying to harmonize.

How about going caroling? In early American history caroling was often a rowdy affair where people would band together and go from house to house banging on pots and pans, trying to get all the neighbors to come along. Then they would sing (and drink) until early in the morning. While we can't recommend this particular variation, you may want to make your caroling livelier by trying to entice your neighbors into joining you, bringing along simple musical instruments, or carrying candles mounted on poles.

I've always wanted a real Yule log. How do you do it?

To carry out this ritual as it used to be done, you need a large, open fireplace and easy access to the woods. First, gather up a special Yule log search party, and then comb the woods for a large, knotty, water-soaked hardwood log. On Christmas morning, make a hot fire with dry kindling and smaller pieces of wood, and top it with the Yule log. As long as the Yule log burns (and you may be able to keep it burning for several days), follow the ancient tradition and ban all nonessential work. When the log finally burns out, save a piece of it to start next year's Yule log.

When we've opened our gifts, Christmas is as good as done with. What are some ways to keep Christmas alive for the rest of the holiday season?

Children, especially, need some way to occupy themselves when the gift exchange is over. After opening your gifts, how about giving a Christmas treat to the birds? Decorate a tree close to your living room window with bird food so the whole family can enjoy watching them feed. If you put out a variety of food, you'll attract more than one kind of bird. Here are some recommendations:

* Unsalted peanuts in shells, strung with heavy-duty thread
* Apple pieces
* Beef suet
* Bread crumbs dipped in peanut butter
* Breadsticks
* Rice cakes
* Popcorn

If your children are at all theatrical, ask them to prepare a skit or play to give the day after Christmas. You can check books out of the library with simple Christmas plays, or let them dream up a simple plot of their own. Encourage them to dress up and add songs.

When the holiday season draws to a close, you might want to have an end-of Christmas ceremony. Gather the family together to take the ornaments off the tree and carefully pack them away. If you have a live tree, replant it outdoors or put it in a sheltered place until the ground thaws. If you have a cut tree, either burn it (carefully) or decorate it with food for the birds. One family explained to us that making a special occasion of ending the holiday "put a seal on Christmas, and promised that it would come again."

Appendix

RESOURCES FOR A SIMPLE CHRISTMAS

✳

✳

✳

✳

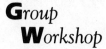

Group **W**orkshop

In this revised edition, we have the pleasure of introducing to you a new resource for your church, business, parents' group, women's group, or other organization. The *Leader's Guide to the Unplug the Christmas Machine Workshop* by Jo Robinson and Jean Staeheli is now available through William Morrow and Company. This guide allows you to convey in a group setting the information contained in this book. In a few hours, participants will be able to take an inventory of their current practices, define their values, create a fantasy celebration, and then combine all their insights into a workable plan for the coming celebration.

Anyone with leadership experience will be able to follow the detailed instructions and put on a successful workshop. The workshop is typically given in one four-hour session, but instructions are given on how to break it up into one-hour segments to be given on four separate days. The guide, which costs $20.00, contains all the material you will need and can be ordered from the publisher or through your local bookstore. (See the order form on page 195.)

About the Appendix

In the remainder of this book, you will find the best ideas we have discovered for simplifying Christmas and making it more enjoyable at the same time. Many of these suggestions have come from the people we have interviewed and who have come to our workshops. Others were inspired by current books and magazines, or descriptions of past Christmases. Whether you decide to adopt any of these suggestions exactly as presented or use them to inspire your own creative thoughts, we hope you will gain a new appreciation for the simple joys of Christmas.

Decorations

Bringing down the boxes of ornaments from the attic, polishing the candlesticks, replacing the burned-out tree lights, and sorting the greens and ribbon for the front door wreath—all of these decorating activities are integral parts of Christmas for most people. Through their own natural beauty and intimate association with happy times, a lighted tree, candles, and all the other beloved objects of the season can transform your everyday surroundings into something magical. No matter how many other things people may want to change about the holiday, very few would eliminate Christmas decorations entirely.

But lots of people would welcome a reduction in the amount of time, effort, and money they spend decorating for the holidays. They want to be able to delight in the physical beauty of Christmas without being preoccupied with the way Christmas looks. On the following pages, you will find simple decorating suggestions that will provide the setting for a wonderful Christmas without overtaxing your energy or pocketbook.

Greens

"It is pleasant to awake on Christmas morning in familiar surroundings, yet made unfamiliar by a green Yuletide welcome."
HOUSE BEAUTIFUL, 1911

Bringing in greens is a wonderful way to transform your everyday environment into a festive one. Even if you do nothing more than highlight greens with an occasional red ribbon or colorful ornament, their appearance is enough to announce that it is Christmas. But besides their beauty, they have other advantages: (1) you can often gather them yourself for nothing, or purchase them at garden shops inexpensively; (2) they have a long and honorable association with Christmas; and (3) you don't have to be an artist to make them look good.

Man-made ornaments didn't become generally available in the United States until the 1870s, so greens were about the only decorations there were. Here are some nineteenth-century ideas to inspire you:

✻ Arrange a combination of ferns, evergreens, and holly berries in a vase, instead of flowers, and use as a table centerpiece.

✻ Place a small stem of holly on each cloth dinner napkin on Christmas Day.

✻ Use holly to decorate your wrapped packages. The plainer the wrapping paper, the better.

✻ Outline doorways, moldings, architectural details and picture frames with evergreen garlands. (This was the classic nineteenth-century treatment.)

✻ Collect dried flowers, weeds, cones, leaves, and corn husks for use in wreaths or table arrangements. Suggestions: goldenrod and milkweed pods dry without special preserving; thistles, leaves, and berries can be preserved by sticking the stems in a solution of one part glycerin (from a drugstore) to two parts water; flowers, such as Queen Anne's lace, can be placed in airtight boxes and surrounded with silica gel until they are completely dried and quite brittle; cones can be left natural, cut in half to reveal their beautiful patterns, glittered, or painted gold and used as accents in wreaths and other arrangements.

If you live in a mild climate, bring in branches of forsythia, cherry, or other flowering trees and force-bloom them in time for Christmas. It was the custom in many European countries to bring the branches inside on St. Barbara's Day, December 4, and try to get them to bloom for Christmas Eve. Any unmarried girl who accomplished this was sure to find a husband before the new year was out.

✳ Decorate any indoor plant or tree that has branches with small ornaments. Small red ribbons on a Norfolk Island pine, masses of white lights on a large jade tree, and a ficus festooned with colorful popcorn and cranberry strings are examples. In addition, dried flower blossoms, nuts (plain or gilded), and raffia ornaments are colorful and light enough for indoor plants.

Although it's fun to look around your house and think of ways to decorate with plants you already have, there is a special pleasure in using traditional greens. Here's a little history on each one.

Mistletoe was a sacred plant with magical properties for ancient European peoples long before its more playful association with Christmas. In medieval Europe, *holly and ivy* were the most important Christmas greens. In the old carol "The Holly and the Ivy" holly represents men and ivy represents women as they argue in fun over which sex is superior. *Rosemary* was prized at Christmas for its pungent scent and its long-lasting leaves. In the Scandinavian countries, *wheat sheaves* were saved from the harvest and mounted on tall poles for good luck during the coming year. In Eastern European countries, *straw* was also placed on tables or on the floor as a reminder of the stable where Jesus was born. *Poinsettias*, now a common Christmas motif, were cultivated by the Aztecs in Mexico, and first incorporated into the Christmas celebration by the Franciscan monks in Mexico in the seventeenth century.

Candles

"If there is a mantel and it is filled with things—off must come the things. When it is as bare as Mother Hubbard's cupboard, bring out all the candlesticks in the house for inspection."
HOUSE BEAUTIFUL, 1908

In addition to greens, candles are a simple and natural way to decorate for Christmas, and if you shop wisely or make your own, they can also be inexpensive. Candles have always been an important part of the winter festival, even predating the Christian celebration itself. In Europe, the lighting of the Christmas Eve candle by the oldest member of the household has been an important ritual for centuries. In Sweden, candles were indispensable to the Lucia Festival, in which the oldest daughter in each family was dressed in white and crowned with a circle of lighted tapers. In the late Middle Ages, pyramids made of tiers of wooden shelves were decorated with candles and carried in processions. In Mexico, candles were put in brown paper bags weighted with sand, and these *luminarias* were used to light the paths of Christmas processions. The Jewish celebration of Hanukkah centers on the ritual of lighting, on successive nights, eight candles held in a candelabrum called a *menorah*. And many Christian families today celebrate Advent by the ceremonious lighting of candles in a special Advent wreath.

But aside from these ritual uses, candles are part of Christmas because people like them. Nothing can make our world into a softer, more beautiful place faster than candles. Recently we visited a house where the only Christmas decorations were masses of candles in different parts of the main room. The electric lights were turned off, and everywhere there was a soft glow. On the mantel were groups of six or seven red votive candles in punch glasses, on the coffee table were several floating candles in glass containers, every windowsill was lit with long bayberry tapers in brass and silver candlesticks, and the buffet table was crowned with a cranberry candle surrounded by a circle of cedar boughs. It was simple and stunning. The hostess told us it was also practical. Candles offer variety, they smell delicious, they are traditional, and the light is so flattering that you can relax about vacuuming and dusting.

When you think about candles, experiment with holders. Some possibilities: wineglasses; cake and muffin tins; trivets; eggcups; soap dishes; clay or plastic plant pots filled with sand, dirt, or gravel. Add small inexpensive mirrors to reflect more light. A glass hurricane-lamp globe can be placed over a candle for a special effect. (And don't forget kerosene lamps themselves. They can be as expensive or inexpensive as you wish, and if you have the kind with a clear glass reservoir, colored lamp oil will brighten your room.)

Aromatic decorations

For many people, nothing is as pleasant or memorable at Christmas as the way it smells. And often what smells good is also beautiful to look at. Here are some simple ways to appeal to the senses:

✳ Pomander balls. Stud a thick-skinned orange with cloves (about one pound of cloves for a dozen oranges). After they have drained for a day on paper towels, roll them in ground spices, such as cinnamon, ginger, and allspice. If you also add ground orrisroot to this mixture, it will act as a fixative and preserve the fragrance longer. You can then use a big needle threaded with ribbon or string to hang the balls, or wrap them with colorful ribbon, or pile them high in decorative bowls and use them in plant arrangements.

✳ Potpourri. Collect broken pieces of herbs, spices, and flowers in pretty glass containers, and decorate them with ribbon, yarn, or small ornaments. Some common garden ingredients are mint, rosemary, roses, thyme, lilac, and lavender. You can also add dried citrus peel and cinnamon sticks. Be sure all the ingredients are absolutely dry to prevent mold, and collect three or four times the amount you want to have when everything has dried and settled. If you keep a lid on the container and only open it occasionally, the fragrance will last longer.

✳ Fresh Fruit. Of course, there are strings of cranberries, but don't forget other winter fruits that can add both aroma and color to Christmas. Red apples can be piled high in baskets or stacked in pyramids in shallow glass containers. Several fresh fruits can be grouped on evergreens, and spread along a mantel or side table and accented with nuts. Citrus fruits, pineapples, apples, and pears are especially suitable.

✳ Simple Smells. In addition, it is easy to arrange cinnamon sticks in shallow trays, or burn incense and pungent candles. And nothing is quite as wonderful as the smell of burning wood if yours is among the eighteen million American households that have fireplaces, or the six million that have wood stoves.

The tree

Although greens and candles and pomander balls can add grace and beauty to your decorating, it's the tree that takes center stage at Christmas. For many people, Christmas *is* the tree, even though it is a relative newcomer to the celebration. It wasn't until Queen Victoria's German husband, Prince Albert, decorated a tree for the royal family in 1848 that the custom caught on in England and America. Now most people can't imagine Christmas without one.

Perhaps the easiest and simplest kind of Christmas tree to have is an artificial one with ornaments permanently attached. This is a boon to many of the older people we have talked to, who find going out and getting a freshly cut evergreen and dragging it back to their apartments more than they can manage. And it may also be the answer for people who live in urban areas where evergreens are in short supply or are quite expensive.

But for many people, a real tree captures best all the good feelings they have about Christmas. Certainly a beautifully conceived and decorated tree is a pleasure, and books and magazines are filled to overflowing with ideas on how to decorate one with ingenuity and taste. But the way a tree looks is only part (if a very important part) of how people feel about it. Most people also respond to the sentimental value of familiar ornaments, whether or not they are beautiful. And they tend to get more enjoyment from the tree if they have had a good time decorating it. A tree decorated by one person spending a lot of time will often have a gratifying artistic unity to it, but a tree that involves the whole family is often more satisfying overall.

It's fun to make the tree a special family tradition, with each person playing an important part. Here are some suggestions for a "family tree":

✳ Assign everyone a task. Many men enjoy taking their kids out to get the tree, but they're not always involved in decorating it. Ask yourself what special job could be done by each family member. Certain ornaments could be reserved for each child to hang; the crowning star or angel could be the privilege of the littlest child, held up by the father. Sometimes, it might make sense to leave the entire decorating to the children and/or the father.

✳ Make getting and decorating the tree a ritual:
Set aside a whole day if possible, which everyone in the family reserves in advance.

If you live near a tree farm, take the children and cut your own. When you get home, warm yourself with hot chocolate before the fire.

Have a tree-trimming party for the neighbors or your extended family. In advance, get the tree settled in the stand, strings of lights in good working order, some unbreakable ornaments for little ones to put on, simple materials for making ornaments if you wish, and good things to eat and drink.

While your family decorates the tree, put your favorite Christmas music on the stereo, serve eggnog, and light the fire and the candles (but not on the tree, of course—candles on a tree are a fire hazard).

∗ Have every member of your family contribute ornaments to the tree. Encourage them to think of found objects or things that are simple to make: paper clip chains, costume jewelry, rickrack, cookie cutters hung with ribbons, small baskets, paper flowers, tinfoil balls, small toys, and wood shavings.

Many families get great satisfaction from having a living tree that is brought inside from year to year, or purchased new every year and then replanted outside. It can be decorated inexpensively and naturally with tangerines, apples, walnuts, dried grasses and flowers, cones, berries, cranberries, and popcorn. You can replant it by digging a hole one and a half times larger than the root mass, lowering it into the hole, loosening (but not removing) the burlap bag that surrounds it, filling the hole with dirt, surrounding the tree with straw or some kind of mulch, and watering well. If you live in a part of the country that gets frost until spring, you will want to dig your hole in November before the ground freezes. When you think about living trees, don't forget that outside trees can be decorated for the animals with strings of popcorn, rice cakes, hard rolls, birdseed, and nuts.

Many of the families we have talked to like to decorate their trees with ornaments that symbolize important family events. If you are interested in this kind of "family history tree," you can do the following:

∗ Give your child, or grandchild, an ornament every Christmas. When the child grows up and celebrates her first Christmas away from home, surprise her by sending a box filled with her own ornaments early in December.

∗ Collect ornaments (or souvenirs that could become ornaments) on your year-round family excursions. When they are all hanging up on the Christmas tree, you will have visual reminders of your travels together.

∗ Encourage your young child to make things to hang on the tree. Even though some contributions (colored paper, ribbons, drawings, cut paper) are used only once, save and label them to show to your child when he or she is grown.

* Choose an ornament each year that represents an important family event—a new baby, a new house, a graduation, a new job.

Music

Brightening your physical environment is one way to change an everyday mood into a festive one, but perhaps nothing can lift your spirits faster than music. All you have to do is hear your favorite Christmas composition or carol, and you are transported back through pleasant memories of the past and filled with the joy and hope of the coming celebration. Even if the tree, the presents, and the big turkey dinner were all taken away, it would still be Christmas—if you had Christmas music.

Owning your own albums is wonderful, but you don't have to be limited by the amount of money you have to spend on them. Most local libraries have a wide selection of Christmas records to choose from, and taking potluck can be an adventure. You never know when you might stumble across a record that will add something new to your enjoyment of the holiday.

You can also make your own music. Regardless of how you sound, singing and playing yourself can give you satisfaction that is hard to surpass.

Caroling is the musical tradition that everyone thinks of first at Christmas. Which of us doesn't have memories of standing outside in the frosty air, raising his voice with others in glorious, out-of-tune song? But aside from providing pleasant memories, caroling has several other advantages:

* People of different ages can enjoy something together, especially if you carol in nursing homes and if your group is composed of both young and old people.
* Caroling reinforces neighborhood unity by giving you a chance to do something nice for neighbors you would not normally see.
* It gets people outside and physically active.
* It provides an important link to the outside for people who are isolated because of age or ill health.
* It doesn't cost anything.

If you would like to go caroling, there are a few things you can do to make it more enjoyable: (1) notify ahead of time the people or institutions (especially nursing homes) you would like to sing for; (2) make sure your singers have copies of the words to more obscure second or third verses; (3) make sure that everyone is dressed warmly enough; (4) have hot drinks available along the way or when you get back home.

But you don't have to leave your house to make your own Christmas music. Many people have told us that getting together to pound the piano and warm up on the guitar is one of the activities they enjoy most at Christmastime. How you sound seems to matter less than the spirit of fun that permeates the music. And, as one professional choir director told us, this is a good way to combat the tendency people have to be spectators at their own celebrations.

Making music at home is also an important way for children to grasp the meaning of the entire Christmas season. Several families we have talked to mark each of the four parts of the holiday—before Christmas, Christmas Eve, Christmas morning, and Epiphany when the Three Kings traveled to Bethlehem to pay homage to the Baby Jesus—with special carols. For example, "Deck the Halls," "Jingle Bells," and "O Come, O Come, Emanuel" can be sung before Christmas; "Silent Night" and "O Little Town of Bethlehem" on Christmas Eve; "Joy to the World" and "Hark! The Herald Angels Sing" on Christmas Day; and "The Twelve Days of Christmas" and "We Three Kings" during Epiphany.

If you want to play or sing Christmas music at home, here are two good resources: *The Oxford Book of Carols* edited by Percy Dearmer (Oxford: Oxford University Press, 1964), which is complete and has creative settings for traditional and nontraditional carols; and *The International Book of Christmas Carols* by Walter Ehret and George K. Evans (Brattleboro, VT: Stephen Greene Press, 1980), which has a wide selection of music, with simple piano arrangements.

Christmas Cards

Christmas cards have been a staple of the celebration for over a hundred years, and many people value them as a good way to stay in touch with those who might otherwise fade from view. But more and more people are questioning the time and expense they require and challenging the unwritten assumption that Christmas wouldn't be Christmas without them.

Ironically, Christmas cards were originally designed to save people work at Christmas. In 1843 Sir Henry Cole commissioned John Calcott Horsley to design a card that would take away the stress of having to write personal letters to all his friends and relatives at Christmas. Cards soon became so successful in England that, as soon as the postal system grew advanced enough to handle the avalanche, everyone started sending them.

Christmas cards caught on in the United States when Louis Prang, a German immigrant lithographer, held an open competition for card artists in 1880 and began producing beautiful cards in great numbers. By the end of the 1880s, Christmas cards were lavish, and sales were in the millions.

In fact, Christmas cards were such an established part of Christmas by the late 1880s that they became a solution to the ever present gift-giving problem. It was considered just as personal to express your feelings for friends through cards as gifts—and it was a lot easier. But cards didn't replace gifts for long. Soon they were being sent *in addition* to gifts, and now many people are trying to find ways to simplify both.

Although lots of people have eliminated Christmas cards altogether, many others are uncomfortable with this abrupt ending of a once-valued tradition. So they are finding ways to modify their every-friend-gets-one card approach by making some modifications:

* Send your cards after Christmas, and make them seasonal cards, rather than Christmas cards. Or send them on Valentine's Day, which is less hectic for you and gives your recipients more time to enjoy them.

* Reduce the number of cards you must purchase, sign, address, and mail by sending them only to people you seldom see.

* Send birthday cards with personal notes in them to people you care about, rather than Christmas cards. While many people expect Christmas cards, they are surprised and delighted when their birthdays are remembered.

* To cut the cost and make your cards more personal, create simple cards by copying one of your children's drawings on a copier. They can also include a seasonal message written by your child.

✳ Instead of sending Christmas cards, write a Christmas letter. This is an easy way for you to share information about your family and saves you from having to write the same letter to several different people. Other members of your family can contribute to the writing or illustrating. (A note on the bottom takes away the impersonal nature of the letter.)

To make your cards more meaningful, you can buy them from a nonprofit organization that supports a cause that you believe in. Examples: UNICEF (333 East 38th Street, New York, NY 10016), the National Wildlife Federation (8925 Leesburg Pike, Vienna, VA 22184), the Fellowship of Reconciliation, an international peace organization (P.O. Box 271, Nyack, NY 10960), or the Sierra Club (730 Polk Street, San Francisco, CA 94109).

If you are a supporter of the arts, you can buy cards produced by local artists. Art museums, speciality shops, art schools, and galleries are good places to find them.

People who are concerned about the environment can purchase cards printed on recycled paper or make cards that double as tree ornaments and won't be tossed away when Christmas is over.

Entertaining

The desire to get together with friends at Christmas is almost universal. We have talked to a few people who confessed they would enjoy a solitary Christmas, but most people envision a celebration filled with friends. They want to share their Christmas pleasures with those whose company they enjoy and feel comfortable in. A women's magazine recently polled its readers and found that they entertain an average of four to nine times during the holiday season. That means that a lot of people are giving thought to hosting dinners, parties, and luncheons.

It also means that a lot of people are trying to entertain on top of already full lives. How can you get together with your friends easily and simply at Christmas, and still get the feelings of fulfillment and closeness to others you want?

One of the most important things you can do for yourself is take the pressure off your own performance. Here are some suggestions to help you shift the emphasis off your role as a cook so you can enjoy a good time with others:

✳ Involve your guests in the preparations of the meal. For example, you could have a "Christmas leftover party," where guests bring leftover stuffing, salad, pie, and so on. Use your imagination to combine these ingredients in new ways. This gives you a chance to try other people's Christmas specialties, and makes the whole group responsible for the results.

✳ Plan a meal that your guests make themselves, such as make-your-own pizza, sandwiches, tacos, or a salad; or divide up the meal so the men make the lasagna and the women make the salad.

✳ Make the process of eating a ritual. Main dishes that lend themselves to ritual are cheese fondue; meat fondue, with chunks of meat fried in hot oil or stock and dipped into a variety of sauces; sausages roasted over the fire; cooked crab, to be cracked and dipped into sauce or melted butter.

✳ Plan a tasting party in which guests provide wine, coffee, cheeses, or other food to share. Here the emphasis is on the variety and quality of the items contributed, and not on your culinary skills, although you might want to provide breads, crackers, or cookies.

✳ Organize a progressive dinner, in which each course is provided by a different household and the entire party moves from one place to another. This works especially well when everyone lives in the same neighborhood or apartment building.

✳ Issue spontaneous invitations so that no one expects a grand performance. A recent study found that the main reason women don't invite their friends to their houses more often is that they are afraid their houses aren't clean enough. As an experiment, you might invite friends over when your house is still a little rough around the edges, just to see what it feels like. If you include children in the invitation, you will change expectations in the direction of a more fun, chaotic, "happy madhouse" atmosphere.

✳ Balance the eating part of the evening with activities that encourage everyone's involvement. (See chapter 9 for suggestions for games and so forth.)

In addition to taking the spotlight off your own performance, you can plan to entertain when you are less busy by having an after-Christmas party, like an Epiphany party on January 6 or an end-of-winter party in

February, when your invitation will come as a welcome break rather than another social obligation to be crowded into an already busy Christmas season.

But whenever you decide to entertain, invite your guests to simpler meals. Instead of having a full-blown sit-down dinner with your best china, consider inviting your friends for brunch, for drinks, for dessert, or even for tea. If you shift the focus slightly away from the food and toward the interaction of the people present, the responsibility for a good time is shared by everyone.

Another way to make entertaining easier, though not cheaper, is to hire help. There are caterers who will prepare and serve the food and clean up afterward. There are people who will clean your house, renew your upholstery, bleach your drapes, rejuvenate your yard, remodel your bathroom, paint your smudgy walls, and deliver your flowers.

Food

It has always been one of the privileges of the Christmas season—a duty, almost—to eat and drink as much as possible. But even if food is an important part of your Christmas, you may have good reasons for wanting to make your food preparation easier. You may be a woman employed outside the home, or a single parent, or tired of starving yourself in January to pay for the sins of December. Or you may simply believe in an ethic of moderation. Here are some suggestions for holiday food that tastes great but will get you out of the kitchen faster.

BASIC FRUIT BREAD

1 LOAF

✳

⅓ cup shortening
⅔ cup sugar
1 teaspoon grated lemon rind
1 to 1½ cups fruit pulp
2 beaten eggs
1¾ cups flour
2¼ teaspoons baking powder
½ teaspoon salt

Blend the shortening, sugar, and lemon rind. Add the fruit pulp and eggs. Mix in the flour, baking powder, and salt. Bake in a greased loaf pan for 1 hour in a 350°F oven. (Note: You may have to slightly increase the amount of flour for very moist fruit pulp.)

Variations: Use cinnamon, orange rind, or rum flavoring in place of lemon. Add ½ cup of nuts, or ¼ cup of dried fruit, such as apricot, or ½ cup of coconut. Fruits and vegetables we have used include banana, applesauce, cranberries, pumpkin, and zucchini.

Your cookies can take on a vast array of sizes and shapes when you invite your baking friends to a "cookie-exchange party." Everyone brings six dozen cookies made with her favorite recipe. They are displayed on a big table and each person chooses the six dozen cookies of her choice. You go with one kind and come home with six different kinds. Here are some quick and delicious cookies you might bring to such a party:

✳ —————————————————————

MERINGUES

3 TO 4 DOZEN

2　*egg whites*
　　Pinch of cream of tartar
½ *cup sugar*

Beat the egg whites and the cream of tartar until foamy. Gradually add the sugar until the mixture holds stiff peaks. Drop by the tablespoon onto a well-greased cookie sheet and bake at 225°F for 50 minutes.

Variations: Add ½ cup of coconut and 1 teaspoon of vanilla for coconut macaroons; add 3 tablespoons of cocoa for chocolate macaroons; or add ½ cup of ground nuts. Experiment with spices such as cinnamon and nutmeg.

But cookies don't always need to be made from scratch. Here are some ways to make good cookies fast:

✳ Buy slice-and-bake cookies and decorate them yourself with walnut halves, candied orange peel, miniature marshmallows, raisins, jams, or your own designs made with tubes of prepared frosting.

✳ For easy gingerbread men, add just enough coffee or rum to a gingerbread mix to moisten it (the batter should be very stiff). Form it into a ball, roll the ball out on a generously floured board, and cut it into shapes with a gingerbread cookie cutter. Bake at 350°F for 10 to 12 minutes.

✳ For easy bar cookies, use a cookie mix and follow the directions

159

on the box for bar cookie variations. To make them festive, add mincemeat, candied fruit, or nuts.

If you find yourself too rushed to make dinner some December evening, consider having a "dipping-into-the-pot" dinner. The idea originated with the Swedish custom of *doppa i grytan*. In Sweden, families gather around the pot, where the Christmas ham or sausage has been simmering for many hours, and dip pieces of heavy rye bread into the broth for a light meal or a prelude to a more sumptuous one. If you don't happen to have a ham or sausage simmering, you can use canned or homemade beef or chicken broth. Augment the meals with hunks of cheese, fruit, and wine.

Don't be afraid to use prepared ingredients in your holiday food. For example:

* Simple marinated vegetables can be made by adding fresh mushrooms and canned pimientos to purchased marinated artichoke hearts. The marinade from the artichokes will be sufficient for all the vegetables.

* For simple hors d'oeuvres, unwrap a block of cream cheese, pour a few tablespoons of soy sauce over it, and surround it with crackers.

* Another simple hors d'oeuvre: Unwrap a block of cream cheese and cover with ½ pound cooked, shelled shrimp. Top with salsa. If desired, garnish with cilantro.

* Canned creamed herring can be purchased in the meat department of your grocery store. Serve it with crackers, canned pickled beets, and dill pickles.

* Don't forget popcorn. Try it flavored with pepper and Parmesan cheese, or drizzled with garlic butter and herbs.

* To serve a delicious sauerkraut side dish, rinse the sauerkraut under running tap water and squeeze out all the moisture. Then sauté it in butter with sliced onions, white or red wine, and caraway seeds.

More ideas for desserts and food preparation:

* For an elegant and different dessert that can be made in minutes, try this recipe:

ALMOND CAKE

1 8-INCH LAYER CAKE

* ───────────────────────────────

1   *stick butter (8 tablespoons)*

½ *cup sugar*

1   *cup canned almond paste (found in the gourmet section of most grocery stores)*

3   eggs
2   tablespoons flour
¼   teaspoon salt
1   teaspoon vanilla
¼   teaspoon almond extract
    Powdered sugar (for dusting)

Cream the butter and sugar together. Add the almond paste and mix well. Add the eggs and beat. Mix in the flour, salt, and flavorings. Pour into an 8-inch cake pan and bake for 45 minutes at 350°F. The cake will be moist.

If you want it to look festive, cut a snowflake pattern from a piece of light cardboard, place it over the top of the cooled cake, and sift powdered sugar lightly over it. The sugar will fall into the holes in your design, and when you lift off the paper, the cake will be decorated with a sugar snowflake design. Refrigerate and serve chilled.

* For another easy dessert, prepared mincemeat mixed with a little brandy or rum (optional) is delicious over vanilla ice cream.

* Many people are finding ways to simplify Christmas Eve dinner, in anticipation of the abundant delights of the next day, by serving soup with fresh bread and fruit. For an easy soup, try this:

*
_____

⅓   cup chopped green onion
3   tablespoons butter or margarine
2½ cups canned chicken broth
2   cups canned pumpkin
    Salt and pepper to taste
2   teaspoons lemon juice
1   teaspoon curry powder
    Nutmeg

CURRIED PUMPKIN SOUP
4 TO 5 SERVINGS

Sauté the onion in the butter until tender. Add the rest of the ingredients (except the nutmeg) and simmer for 10 minutes. Sprinkle with the nutmeg and serve.

* Restrict your Christmas baking to the week before Christmas to keep your time in the kitchen and the amount you eat under control. An added benefit is that you won't get tired of Christmas specialties.

* Many people discover that some part of their holiday food preparations falls into the "excessive" category. Consider making half the number of cookies you usually bake, or eliminating the third pie at Christmas dinner.

* By accepting the sometimes less-than-perfect results of your children's cooking and welcoming the participation of your husband, you can spend less time in the kitchen doing less complicated dishes. Establish food traditions that depend on the involvement of every family member. Find out what your husband and children would like to make, and let them make it—year after year.

* Your children may be able to do more to help you than you think. Consider asking children six to ten years old to help in the following ways:

Making place cards for the dinner table
Setting the table
Measuring baking ingredients and pouring them into the mixer
Simple chopping, peeling, slicing, and grating
Icing and decorating cookies
Running errands
Answering the phone and taking messages
Forming cookies on a cookie sheet
Washing dishes and cleaning up

* Even if you can't afford caterers who cook, serve, and clean up after special parties, you may find that buying baked goods or buffet meats and cheeses from a delicatessen is worth the extra expense.

* Do you know of a lonely friend or neighbor, perhaps a grandmother, who would welcome the hustle and bustle of your kitchen for a little while? She can help you make cookies then take some home for herself.

Healthy food

Every year I engage in this gargantuan battle between Thanksgiving and New Year's. Here I am in the middle of this diet, and along comes Christmas. And the fudge. And I eat too much and am defeated once again. So I starve myself in January to make up for it.

Does this sound like you? If so, you have lots of company. This roller coaster ride of overindulging and then starving oneself is a well established Christmas tradition. Historically, it was less than a century ago that our forebears saved up treasured amounts of coffee, sugar, and white flour to add something special to the sit-down feast that would break up the cold, dark, hardworking monotony of winter. During most of our history, the majority of people have looked forward to Christmas as a hard-earned celebration of abundance. It is only recently, with our easy prosperity,

that Christmas has slipped over the line and become, for many, a celebration of overabundance.

Many of us may not realize how familiar and comfortable this cycle
has become. We might not be able to enjoy the overeating of December
without the security of knowing that we will have to "buckle down" in
January. And conversely, we might not be ready to get serious about our
health habits in January without the fresh guilt of our indiscretions to
spur us on.

This is not to say that this pattern is written in stone. It may be
familiar to you, and it may be sanctioned by our culture, but it is not
an inevitable part of Christmas. And, ultimately, it may not be the
healthiest way to live. This cultural overabundance/scarcity pattern mirrors the personal binge/starve cycle that can be so detrimental to the
development of healthy eating patterns.

In order to find out how to smooth out the bump in the yearly cycle
and eat well all year, we talked to Herman M. Frankel, M.D., director
of the Portland Health Institute. Dr. Frankel, a nationally recognized
physician, and three-time national chairman of The Obesity Foundation,
has many years of experience in helping people change life-style patterns
that are no longer working for them.

If you are ready to eat as healthfully in December as you do in June,
Dr. Frankel has the following suggestions:

1 Eat starchy foods During the holiday season, as well as during the
rest of the year, it is important to get most of your calories from foods
that are high in complex carbohydrates such as breads, cooked grains,
pasta, fruit, and starchy vegetables such as potatoes, yams, and squash.
One hundred calories of starch will deposit less fat in your body than
one hundred calories of fat, and will, at the same time, make deposits
into your energy stores in the form of glycogen (the form in which human
beings store carbohydrates). The complement to this idea is to consume
as little fat, sugar, and alcohol as is comfortable for you.

2 Eat often, at the first sign of hunger For many people, this means
every two or three hours throughout the waking day. You can think of
this as compulsive-eating *prevention*. By continually replenishing your
stores of glycogen, you are protecting yourself from feeling famished. At
the same time, you are ensuring that when you do sit down to Christmas

dinner you will feel like making healthy food choices, instead of careening out of control with the hungries. People who eat frequently will very seldom binge.

3 Eat before going out When you've accepted an invitation to a holiday party, eat a piece of bread or fruit before you leave home. If you begin the social occasion with a comfortable feeling of fullness, you will be less likely to make frequent forays into the canapés.

4 Allow yourself to enjoy special foods of the season Many people want to have the pleasure of eating festive food that is special to the season. If this is true for you, it will be easier to be moderate if, ahead of time, you mentally rehearse taking one small piece of fruitcake, or only one or two Christmas cookies instead of a bunch. Preparing in advance, by visualizing yourself making healthy choices, can help you participate in the festive atmosphere without overdoing it or feeling deprived.

5 Take care of yourself Be sure to schedule time for yourself, even in the midst of the Christmas craziness. You will find it much easier to maintain healthy eating habits if you are getting enough sleep, having enough time alone, keeping to an exercise routine, and resting when you are tired.

6 Continue doing what works for you If you exercise, then you are already doing one of the most important things you can do for your health. By continuing to walk, bicycle, work out, or swim during the Christmas season, you will help yourself deal better with stress, and give your body the messsage that it can keep on burning fat. If you are one of those few people who keeps food diaries for your own information, continue to do so, and you will be able to round out your understanding of your own habits during a time when the temptations to eat are stronger.

7 Seek and give social support Remember that if you are trying to cut down on fats, sweets, and alcohol, you have lots of company. Many, many other people are trying to do the same thing. Nowadays, a "no thank-you" at the dessert tray hardly raises an eyebrow, and turning down a drink is often greeted by admiration. Also, you may be gratified to find out how much appreciation you'll receive when you bring healthful, low-fat dishes to the holiday table.

The Christmas season is an opportunity to express and celebrate a wide array of values that add meaning to our lives. Eating is only one way we take pleasure in the season. There are so many other ways to celebrate. We can reach out to someone who needs a kind word. We can spend time reading to our children. We can enjoy an hour or two sitting by the fire, absorbing the beauty of a freshly decorated tree. We can glory in the power of music to move us. And we can feel good about the way our seasonal habits continue to move us toward health.

To help you see that it is possible to prepare festive food that is delicious and low in fat, we have included recipes for a few of the favorite dishes from the Portland Health Institute. Please feel free to write to Portland Health Institute, 9045 SW Barbur Boulevard, Portland, OR 97219, if you would like more information on how to develop and maintain the habits that will enable you to live well and healthfully during the holiday season, and throughout the rest of the year.

Festive, low-fat dessert ideas

✳ Buy an angel food cake. Slice it and serve it with fresh fruit or a fruit sauce and sweetened, nonfat yogurt on top.

✳ Serve low-fat ice cream or frozen yogurt with a sprinkling of crushed candy cane on top. Add a small candy cane for decoration.

✳ Try this delicious, nonfat, red-and-green dessert. Peel, cut in half, and core a few ripe winter pears. Simmer 15 to 20 minutes in sweetened-to taste, condensed cranberry juice. (Reconstitute frozen cranberry juice with one half the recommended amount of water.) Serve the pears warm or cold in the juice, decorated with sprigs of fresh mint. (Nondieters can add a dollop of whipped cream.)

Low-fat recipes

Christmas is a time when people do a lot of buffet entertaining. The following six recipes for dips and spreads are very low in fat and can be served with bread, crackers, and vegetables. Many guests will appreciate having a low-fat option in a season replete with eggnog and fudge.

HUMMUS

✳

Hummus is a traditional Middle Eastern dish that is customarily full of olive oil. This version is almost fat-free.

1 15-ounce can garbanzo beans, rinsed and drained (2 cups cooked beans)
   Juice of 1 lemon
3 cloves of garlic, peeled and minced
⅓ cup nonfat yogurt
1 teaspoon salt

Fresh, chopped parsley or scallion (for garnish)

Blend all the ingredients in a food processor until desired consistency is reached. You may add more yogurt if needed. Serve on bread or as a dip for vegetables.

Variations: Add any of the following spices to taste: cumin, turmeric, curry powder, chile pepper, or prepared picante sauce. You may also substitute rice vinegar or seasoned rice vinegar for the lemon juice. If you don't mind the extra fat, you may add one or two tablespoons of tahini (sesame paste) in place of some of the yogurt. The hummus may be garnished with fresh, chopped parsley or fresh, chopped scallion.

TOMATO BUTTER

✳

1 15-ounce can whole, peeled tomatoes, including the liquid
2 cloves of garlic, peeled and minced
2 tablespoons seasoned rice vinegar
1 teaspoon dried basil
¼ teaspoon black pepper

Mix all the ingredients together in a saucepan and bring to a boil. Reduce the heat and simmer, uncovered, until blended and thickened (about 45 minutes to 1 hour). May be served as a spread on bread, or in place of regular tomato sauce in pizza and lasagne.

RED BEAN DIP

✳

1 15-ounce can red beans, rinsed and drained
2 tablespoons tomato sauce
2 tablespoons mild picante sauce
2 tablespoons fresh, chopped cilantro (coriander)
2 cloves of garlic, peeled and minced
   Salt to taste

Simmer all the ingredients in a saucepan for 10 minutes. Serve as a spread for bread, or with tortilla chips, or as a filling for tortillas.

Note: You may make your own low-fat tortilla chips by cutting corn or whole wheat tortillas into bite-sized triangles, spreading them on a baking sheet, and baking them at 325°F for 20 minutes until crisp but not brown.

✳ ————————————————————

EGGPLANT DIP (BABA GHANNOUJ)

MAKES 1 TO 2 CUPS

1 *large eggplant*
   Juice of 1 large lemon
3 *large cloves of garlic, peeled and minced*
⅔ *cup tomato paste*
1 *teaspoon salt*
¼ *teaspoon chile pepper*

   Fresh, chopped parsley (for garnish)

Cut the tip off the eggplant. Bake at 350°F for 30 minutes until soft all over and partly collapsed. Cool. Remove the peel. Blend in a food processor until smooth.

Mix in the other ingredients. Chill for 2 to 3 hours.

Garnish with fresh, chopped parsley. May be served as a dip for vegetables or a spread for bread.

✳ ————————————————————

YOGURT CHEESE

2 CUPS

1 *quart nonfat yogurt*

Spoon the yogurt into a strainer (or cotton cloth or cheesecloth) and allow it to drain for 6 hours or more. The solid product may be used in place of cream cheese or mayonnaise, or when lightly whipped, in place of sour cream. You may use the drained liquid in baking bread, in soup, or when cooking rice.

Variations: There are many possibilities for flavorings:

To make a bread spread to replace mayonnaise, add 2 cloves of garlic, minced; 1 teaspoon Dijon mustard; and salt and pepper to taste.

To make a spread to eat alone on bread, add 2 cloves of garlic, minced; 1 tablespoon dried herbs, such as oregano, thyme, basil, parsley, coriander, or dill; 1 tablespoon seasoned rice wine vinegar; and 2 tablespoons grated Parmesan cheese.

To make a topping for Mexican dishes, add ½ cup mild picante sauce.

To make a tartar sauce for fish, add the juice of half a lemon; 1 clove of garlic, minced; 2 tablespoons tomato sauce; and salt and pepper to taste; *or* 3 tablespoons low-fat Thousand Island dressing.

To make a dessert topping (for angel food cake and fruit, for example), add 1 tablespoon honey, ½ teaspoon ground cinnamon, and a dash of nutmeg, *or* 2 tablespoons reduced-sugar jam.

SKORDALIA

MAKES APPROXIMATELY
4 CUPS

✳ ———————————————————————

4   *cups peeled, cooked baking potatoes, cut in chunks*
1½ *cups nonfat plain yogurt*
6   *cloves of garlic, peeled and minced*
1   *to 2 teaspoons salt*
1   *teaspoon lemon juice*
1   *tablespoon fresh, chopped parsley*

Blend all the ingredients in a food processor until smooth. May be served with bread as a spread.

We would like to offer two additional low-fat recipes here that will help you survive the holiday season with your figure intact. The first is for a lentil soup that is delicious and easy to prepare. Nothing warms you up on a cold winter day like a hearty soup. Make it ahead and keep it in the freezer to serve on one of those days when you want to relax and enjoy the company of family and friends. The second recipe is for a low-fat turkey stuffing and gravy. With turkey being naturally low in fat, when the stuffing and gravy are also low in butter and oil, the entire meal stays within healthy eating guidelines.

LENTIL SOUP

MAKES 8 SERVINGS

✳ ———————————————————————

1   *package dried lentils (about 3 cups)*
4   *cans chicken stock (14½ ounces each)*
2   *medium potatoes, peeled and sliced*
1   *large carrot, sliced*
1   *large onion, chopped*
1   *large can whole, peeled tomatoes*
2   *large cloves of garlic, peeled and minced*
1   *teaspoon dried basil*
½   *teaspoon salt*
½   *teaspoon pepper*
⅓   *cup seasoned rice wine vinegar*

Combine all the ingredients and simmer for 45 minutes.

2 *egg whites or egg substitute equivalent*
12 *ounces dried bread crumbs*
3 *cups chicken broth*
½ *pound mushrooms, sliced without stems*
2 *large yellow onions, coarsely chopped*
2 *stalks celery, sliced*
½ *tablespoon ground sage*
½ *tablespoon poultry seasoning*
2 *small cans sliced water chestnuts*
½ *cup raisins*
   Salt and pepper to taste

Work the egg whites or egg substitute into the bread crumbs with your hands.

In a saucepan, heat the chicken broth until simmering. Add the mushrooms, vegetables, and seasonings. Simmer until the vegetables are tender.

Pour the broth and vegetables into the bread crumb mixture, and when cool enough, mix well with your hands, adding the water chestnuts and raisins. Salt and pepper the stuffing to taste.

This stuffing may be stuffed into a turkey or baked by itself as a separate dish.

✳

After the turkey is fully cooked, pour off the pan juices, skim off the fat, and add any or all of the following to taste: lemon juice, plum jam, soy sauce, salt and pepper. The gravy may be thickened with cornstarch. (Mix 3 tablespoons of cornstarch with 5 tablespoons of cold water and blend thoroughly. Pour the gravy juices into a saucepan and heat slowly. As the gravy heats, add the cornstarch mixture and stir constantly. The gravy will begin to thicken as it is stirred.)

Gifts

Of all our modern Christmas traditions, gift giving seems to take the most time, money, and energy. It's not uncommon for people to spend hundreds of dollars and weeks of effort on this one part of Christmas alone. Although few people want to banish gifts altogether, most of them are looking for ways to make the ritual more enjoyable and less of a strain. Here you will find money-saving gift ideas, time-saving gift ideas, alternative gift ideas, and alternative gift sources.

Saving money

Making your own gifts, of course, can save you a lot of money. If you have the time, talent, and energy to devote to a homemade Christmas, there are many wonderful resources to choose from.

However, like many of the people we talk to, you may have as little extra time as money. But even if you buy most of your gifts, there are still ways to cut down on the expense:

✳ If you take a predetermined amount of money out of the bank before you go shopping and declare your credit cards and checks off limits, you will not only save on the high cost of credit, but you will probably make better spending decisions.

✳ Be on the lookout for special sales. For example, stores are fiercely competitive with their brand-name toys, so be sure to do some comparison shopping. You may find the same toy for 25 percent less at another store. And if you're shopping for small home appliances, look for rebates. There are many more of them in December than during the rest of the year.

✳ If you want to save money on gifts, you don't have to look further than your favorite cookbook. The traditional candies, cookies, and fruit bread are always appreciated, but consider making pasta, pesto, herb vinegars, herb bouquets, holiday or interesting breads, chutney, champagne jelly, citron, smoked fish, cheese balls, snack mixes, tea blends, coffee blends, your own mustard.

✳ Tempt fate. Buy your gifts and tree right before Christmas to take advantage of last-minute price-slashing.

✳ Buy inexpensive gifts and let your presentation turn them into elegant ones. For example, to dress up your food gifts, buy a simple basket with an open weave and thread red ribbon through the holes. Wrap the goodies in colored cellophane, arrange them artfully in the basket, and add a handsome card. This way, a dozen cookies can be transformed into a beautiful gift.

✳ Give alternative gifts. For example, call up a friend you don't see often and set a firm date to spend time together instead of exchanging wrapped presents. Or have a recycled Christmas, where each family member chooses something he or she already owns to pass on to another. Or shop at thrift stores or garage sales. (Save this idea for sympathetic family members.)

The cost of mailing gifts can be a significant factor in your overall gift expenses. Here are some ways to trim this hidden expense:

✳ Make sure that you are mailing your packages by the most economical method. You may save plenty of dollars. The best way to get current information is to call your post office and other mail services and ask them to send you a copy of their rate charts.

✳ Think "lightweight" when you are making up your gift list for faraway relatives. A two-pound package might cost $2.85 to mail by parcel post and a fifteen-pound package up to $19.00. Some suggestions: jewelry, photographs, prints, pens, pocketknives, posters, paperback books, tea, herbs, watches, lingerie, silk scarves, records, cassette tapes, calendars, magazine subscriptions, money, memberships, gift certificates.

You can also save money on gift wrapping. Here are some ideas:

✳ Take along your pocket calculator when you buy your wrapping supplies. There may be a great difference in price among products of similar quality. You may save as much as one dollar per package. In general, it's best to buy 125-foot rolls of ribbon, large tubes of gift wrap, and strapping tape that meets postal service standards but does not exceed them (unless you are sending especially heavy packages).

✳ Tie your packages with colorful yarn. It's less expensive than ribbon and does not crumple in the mail. If you buy the yarn in the arts and crafts section rather than the gift wrap department, you can save even more money.

✳ If you are superorganized, buy your supplies for the future during post-Christmas sales. And if you're really cutting corners, iron last year's wrapping paper and ribbon and use them again.

✳ Forget kraft (plain brown) outer wrap and mailing labels on your boxes and save yourself both time and money. The postal service and UPS prefer unwrapped packages sealed with strapping tape and with addresses written directly on the box.

Saving time

When you add up all the time you spend thinking of gifts, shopping for them, making them, gift wrapping them, boxing them for the mail, and hauling them to the post office, you probably have at least a week of concentrated effort. And if you make most of your gifts, you can triple that figure.

If you have the time to relax and enjoy all the details, gift giving can be the best part of Christmas. But if you have to squeeze all those chores into an already-full schedule, the pressure can cancel out the joy.

Here are some ways to spend less time on the mechanical aspects of giving:

✳ Give gift certificates, season tickets, movie tickets, magazine subscriptions (if you didn't send away for the subscriptions soon enough for a copy to arrive on Christmas, wrap up the current issue along with a note), or memberships. These gifts can often be taken care of with one phone call.

✳ Make your gift a tradition. Send the same thing each year and eliminate the time spent searching for the perfect gift. If people enjoy your gift and can count on it year after year, it becomes an important part of the holiday season. Some suggestions: a yearly renewal of a favorite magazine, a box of nuts or top-quality produce, season tickets to a favorite concert series.

✳ Give specialty food products delivered by mail.

✳ Eliminate time-consuming trips to the post office: have the UPS pick up your packages.

✳ If you mail your packages, plan your visits to the post office for the least busy hour, 10–11 A.M., and aim for Thursday, often the slowest day of the week.

✳ Do all your shopping through a book club or in one trip to a bookstore where you will find books to interest every person on your list. (Also, books can be easily slipped into mailers, eliminating the need for more elaborate packaging.)

✳ Stockpile your gifts and wrap them all at once. Set up an efficient wrapping center and wrap everything with the same paper and ribbon. Before you begin, be sure you have scissors, transparent tape, wrapping paper, tissue paper, gift cards (bought or homemade), boxes, and strapping tape. Get the whole family to help.

✳ Shop in stores that offer to wrap and mail your gifts.

✳ Buy colorful Christmas boxes, tie with ribbon, and skip the wrapping paper.

✳ Buy one big gift for an entire family rather than one for each individual and save time on the brainstorming, shopping, wrapping, and mailing.

✳ And the potentially biggest time and money saver of all: shop by catalogue. In recent years you have probably noticed a big increase in the number of Christmas catalogues that find their way into your mailbox. Now you can buy everything from diamonds to rubber boots without leaving home. In many cases you can call a toll-free number, place your order, read off your credit card number, and have the packages delivered to your door or, better yet, right to the recipient. You really *can* do all your Christmas shopping in a matter of hours, while taking advantage of direct mail savings at the same time. You will also be able to make better choices because you can shop without pressure, and you will find it easier to keep track of the total bill and reconsider if you exceed your overall limit.

Gift catalogues

When you shop through catalogues, there are a few things to keep in mind. Many businesses will not process your order until your check clears, and that may take two weeks. To avoid delays, send money orders or pay with a credit card. Second, when you send along enclosures (checks or coins) be sure to indicate that in writing so they will not be overlooked. Third, date your letter and keep a photocopy or carbon in case there are any problems. Fourth, when your package arrives, examine the contents immediately to make sure the items have not been damaged and that you got what you ordered.

If you'd like a list of over 250 catalogues, send away for the *Great Catalog Guide,* a publication issued annually by the Direct Marketing Association (DMA). To get a copy, send a three-dollar check or money order to: Great Catalog Guide, Direct Marketing Association, 11 West 42nd Street, P.O. Box 3861, New York, NY 10163–3861.

Alternative gift ideas

Many people are feeling a need to find alternatives to commercial gift giving. The alternative gift ideas in this section cover a lot of ground. They include classic gift ideas that are often overlooked in the scramble for this year's hottest fads. There are also gifts of service, easy homemade gifts requiring little time or talent, unusual store-bought gifts, and gift ideas to spark your imagination.

IDEAS FOR CHILDREN

When you shop for children, look for toys that are durable, washable, have no sharp points or edges, encourage peaceful, creative play, and continue to be useful even when some of the pieces get lost.

Buy safe toys. Check for the mark "ASTMF:963," indicating that the toy conforms to the voluntary safety standards established by the toy industry. If you have more questions about toy safety, call the U.S. Consumer Product Safety Commission's toll-free hot line: (800) 638-2772.

You will find that most toys are labeled according to age range, but toy experts say that most manufacturers "label up," which means they recommend that toys be used by slightly older children than is truly appropriate. For a more realistic estimate, take six months off the lower age number and a year off the top.

The suggestions that follow are for a mixture of simple, classic toys and more novel gift ideas.

∗ Infants

Cloth blocks
Clutch ball
Crib gym
Mobile (The windup kind that plays music is more entertaining.)
Rubber teether
Baby mirror (made of unbreakable steel)
Plastic key ring
Stuffed animal
Bristle Blocks (Infants like to chew on them. Older ones can stick them together.)
Suction toy for the high chair

∗ One- to three-year-olds

Tiny nesting boxes
Appliance box with doors and window cut in it
Box of gummed labels
Box of adhesive bandages
Real flashlight and batteries
Collection of improvised bath toys (a plastic funnel, a turkey baster,

an empty plastic shampoo bottle, plastic measuring spoons and cups, etc.)

Piggy bank with starter money

Homemade Play-Doh

Hinged objects

Pull toy

Riding toy

Stuffed animal

Wooden stringing beads

Blocks

Ball

Milk bottle carrier

Stacking toy

Pounding toy

Shape sorter

Truck

Car

Doll

Plastic building blocks (large)

Wooden knob puzzle

Modeling clay

Gift-wrapping ideas for toddlers: tie bells to ribbon and make the paper easy to unwrap.

✳ Four- to six-year-olds

Deck of cards

Homemade balance beam

Map of the town with the child's own house, school, Mommy's and Daddy's offices, church, library, zoo, etc. highlighted

Old suitcase filled with play clothes (veils, scarves, belts, hats, a nurse's hat, an apron, a tie, etc.)

Costume jewelry

Ticket for a ride on a real train

Banner with the child's name on it

Office supplies in a homemade executive kit

Art supplies

Strong magnet

Magnifying glass

Bird feeder

Magazine subscription (see page 177)

Sewing kit

Harmonica, drum set, or slide flute

Real brass bell

Simple book about the child that you wrote and illustrated

Real stethoscope (available at medical supply houses)

Puzzle (up to a hundred pieces)

Play people

Dolls and dollhouse

Building blocks (small)

Paint and easel

Simple board or card game

Picture book

Record

Cassette tape

Tricycle or bike

Slinky

✳ Grade-school children

Ticket to a favorite sporting event

Real sports equipment

Book of movie tickets

Homemade sewing kit

Embroidery hoop, material, needles, and embroidery thread

Leaf press

Scrapbook

Music lessons

Simple instrument

Calendar

Science kit

Knitting needles and yarn

Crochet hook and yarn

Real cooking equipment

Video or computer game
Science project
Aquarium
Weather equipment
Hand-held calculator
Shares of stock
One-egg chick incubator (available in science stores)
Simple camera and photo album
Pocket Tinker Toys
Three-dimensional puzzle
Coin or stamp collecting album
Magazine subscription

These are four children's magazines that received high marks from librarians and teachers.

Cricket has been called "the only truly literary magazine for children ages 6–14." Its editorial board includes Isaac Bashevis Singer, Trina Schart Hyman, Lloyd Alexander, Virginia Hamilton, and Nancy Larrick. *Cricket* features articles, stories, poems, and illustrations by internationally known children's authors and illustrators. For twelve issues, send $29.97 to: *Cricket*, P.O. Box 52961, Boulder, CO 80321; or call (800) BUG-PALS.

Ladybug is a new magazine for toddlers, preschoolers, and beginning readers from the publishers of *Cricket*. Each issue has thirty-six pages of easy picture stories, songs, poems, rhymes, and a more challenging read-aloud story. The magazine is beautifully written and based on sound educational principles. For eight issues for $14.97, call (800) BUG-PALS.

Ranger Rick's Nature Magazine features activities and information to help children ages five to twelve enjoy nature and appreciate the need for conservation. For twelve issues, send $15 to: Ranger Rick, National Wildlife Federation, 8925 Leesburg Pike, Vienna, VA 22184; or call (800) 432-6564.

Stone Soup is a collection of stories, poems, book reviews, and drawings done by children ages six to thirteen for children of the same ages. For a subscription, send $23 to: *Stone Soup*, Children's Art Foundation, P.O. Box 83, Santa Cruz, CA 95063.

✳ **Teenagers**

Donation to a favorite charity (Save the Whales, etc.)
UNICEF concert records
Music lessons
Book of movie tickets
Telephone credit
Session with a cosmetic expert
Credit at a bookstore
Credit at a record store
Photography lessons
Sports lessons
Cooking lessons
Blank book for a journal
Book on drawing, pencils, and art paper
Special lunch or dinner at a nice restaurant
Calligraphy pen and an instruction book
Record (Get suggestions about a favorite recording star.)
Cassette tape for the car
Dictionary
Furniture for the teenager's room
Sheets or a down comforter
Sports equipment
Camping equipment
Subscription to a magazine in a prospective career field, or one of general interest
Invitation to a ballet, play, or concert
Ten dollars in quarters for video games
Shares of stock
Money

GIFT IDEAS FOR ADULTS

If you would like to give out-of-the-ordinary gifts, shop at out-of-the ordinary stores and sources, like:

Marine supply stores
Government surplus stores

Import stores
Restaurant supply stores
Antique stores
Museum shops
Arts and crafts galleries
Damaged-freight stores
Stationery stores
Classified ads
Garage sales
Plant nurseries
Hardware stores
Health food stores

Further a fantasy—give a subscription to a magazine or a book on a secret ambition (for example: *Writer's Digest* for a budding writer, or a book on inventions for a would-be inventor).

Telephone credit

Collection of favorite family recipes

Collection of small things that the person habitually loses (pens, safety pins, scissors, Scotch tape, etc.)

Address and phone number of a lost friend or relative

One-hour body massage

Offer to baby-sit for a weekend in the person's house

Complete emergency dinner for the freezer

Saturday work party for an older relative

Cater to a secret indulgence—a subscription to a movie magazine for someone who buys them only on the sly, a big hunk of quality French baking chocolate

Collection of traditional holiday recipes for a grown-up son or daughter

Your family genealogy

Enlarged pictures from old negatives

Catalogue from a local community college plus money for the course of the person's choice

Classical Christmas record

Copy of this book

Weather equipment

Calligraphy pens plus an instruction book

Professional chef's equipment

Specialty food from your part of the country

Family magazine subscription

Load of firewood

Armload of greens

A gift for all your friends with young children: a Christmas party for their children the Saturday before Christmas. They can drop the kids off and have three or four precious hours to shop, wrap, bake, and decorate. You may want to help the children make Christmas cards for their parents; wrapping paper with shelf paper, tempera paint, and potato-block prints; or salt-dough ornaments.

* Gift Ideas for Men (because so many people find them harder to shop for)

Photography or darkroom equipment

Season pass to a favorite sport

Traditional holiday food from his childhood

For a sailor: marine maps

For a hunter: topographical maps

Binoculars

Bird or plant identification book

Subscription to a magazine

One free music lesson on the instrument of his choice

One free flying lesson

Ski lift tickets

Professional chef's equipment

Cookbook

Backpacking equipment

Deluxe first-aid kid for boat, camper, car, or backpacking trips

Gardening book

Outdoor plant

One night (with you) in a hotel

Pasta machine

Sausage stuffer and sausage cookbook

Japanese saws and knives

Pruning equipment
His horoscope
Telescope
Star chart
Book about space
Plastic raft
Ticket for a white-water rafting trip
Print for his office
Gift certificate at a stereo store
Coupon good for an absolutely free weekend somewhere
Enlarged photo of the house where he spent his childhood
Microscope
Horseback-riding lessons
Tennis lessons
Case of tennis balls

✳ Gift Ideas for Older Folks

Take them Christmas shopping
Run errands for them
Have a housecleaning or repair party
Invite them to your house for singing or cookie baking
Set a monthly library or shopping and lunch date
For people with poor eyesight:
    Playing cards with jump numbers
    Large-type books
    The large-type edition of *The New York Times*
    Volunteer to read to them
    Books on tape

IDEAS FOR A FAMILY

If you pick gifts the whole family can enjoy, you will not only simplify your shopping, but help bring that family closer together.

✳ Inexpensive gifts

Two decks of cards and a book of card game rules
Classic board game they don't have and might enjoy
Five-hundred-piece jigsaw puzzle

Three-dimensional puzzle
Badminton set
Magazine subscription
Inner tubes
Sled
Soccer ball
Basketball hoop
Dictionary
Globe
Dwarf fruit tree

✳ More expensive family gifts

Cider press
Food dehydrator
Ice-cream maker
Pasta machine
Telescope
Binoculars
Microscope
Archery equipment
Grain mill
Ski lift tickets

EASY HOMEMADE GIFTS

Many people want to give homemade gifts but don't feel they have the time and/or talent to do the conventional holiday crafts. Here are some gifts that require few special skills and can be as simple or elaborate as you choose to make them:

Special family blend tea and coffee

Buy several of your favorite tea or types of coffee beans in bulk. Come home and experiment with different blends. Call the family in for a taste test and have everyone vote for his or her favorite. The winner is your "Family Blend." Make up a big batch, scoop it into bags, and tie them with ribbons. (Do you have extra time? Design family labels.)

Cracked nuts

If you live in a part of the country where nuts are plentiful, give your friends sacks of cracked nuts. Buy them in bulk in a produce store, or look for a you-pick-it farm in the classified section of your newspaper. Bring the nuts home and crack them in front of the fire. Have little children search for shells in the pile of shelled nuts. Scoop them into sacks and tie with ribbons, or deliver in a woven basket. (These make wonderful early Christmas gifts.)

Roasted nuts

Buy or gather almonds, hazelnuts, cashews, and/or filberts. After shelling them, spread them on a cookie sheet, sprinkle with salt, and bake in a 350°F oven for 5 to 20 minutes depending on size. Deliver them in small baskets, pottery, or plastic sacks with ribbon.

Family cookbook (requires advance planning)

Send a photocopied letter to all your family members asking them for a favorite recipe in their own careful handwriting. Ask them to write on the same sheet of paper a little about the recipe (for example, its history or an amusing anecdote). When you have a collection of recipes, photocopy the original letters. (If you are pressed for time, look for a copier that collates and staples.) The layout can be as simple or as elaborate as you care to make it. This gift will be appreciated by friends as well as family.

Family calendar

Send a photocopied letter to all your relatives asking them for their birth dates, their anniversaries, and the dates of any historic family events (for example, the birth dates of important ancestors, dates when they immigrated or made important moves, and so on). When you have the responses, buy a blank calendar at a stationer's and enter all the events. Take the completed calendar to a printer and have it reproduced. (For a more elaborate production, add historic or current family photographs to the calendar, but plan on paying for a more expensive printing process.)

Family tree

Make an up-to-the-minute family tree complete with birth dates, current addresses, and phone numbers. If you have no drawing skills, simply supply the data in chart form. But if you are artistic, enter the information on a big family tree.

The gift of spring

Give the gift of springtime: a pot of blooming narcissus. (You have to start about two months ahead of time for this one.) Directions for forcing them to bloom: Fill a shallow container with rocks or decorative pebbles and add water until it reaches just below the surface. Set the bulbs on the gravel and add more pebbles to hold them upright. Set the container next to a window, away from direct heat. As the leaves appear, rotate the container so the bulbs will grow evenly. The flowers will bloom in four to six weeks and will last two weeks at room temperature. (The bulbs cannot be repotted.)

Alternative gift sources

The following nonprofit organizations make part of their income by selling Christmas gifts to the public. When you buy gifts from these agencies, the profit goes to benefit their causes. We describe them in sufficient detail so that you can decide which ones you wish to support with your Christmas dollars.

Koinonia Farm

This group is committed to living out the radical teachings of Jesus— peace, human kindness, and simplicity. Part of its support comes from the sale of quality pecan and peanut products. For a catalogue, write to Koinonia Farm, Route 2, Americus, GA 31709. The group will also be glad to send you more information on its life and work.

Sales Exchange for Refugee Rehabilitation Vocations (SERRV)

SERRV, Self-Help Handcrafts, a forty-year-old, not-for-profit ecumenical program of the Church of the Brethren, imports and markets crafts from more than forty-five developing nations. The crafts are purchased from approximately two hundred cooperatives, democratically organized groups and socially responsible crafts producers. SERRV assists these third world artisans by paying a just price for their products, by advancing payment to allow purchase of raw materials, by assisting with product design, and by providing grants.

SERRV's sales are achieved principally through wholesale and consignment sales to three thousand church and community groups throughout the United States. SERRV also markets through its own stores in New York and Maryland, its own retail catalogue, and catalogues of other nonprofit organizations. To become involved with the SERRV resale program, send $3 for an information packet containing a wholesale catalogue (designed for church groups and retail outlets), or request a free direct-mail catalogue for individual ordering. Write to: SERRV, Self-Help Handcrafts, 500 Main Street, New Windsor, MD 21776; or call (800) 423-0071.

SELFHELP Crafts of the World

SELFHELP, a nonprofit program, helps low-income people in developing countries earn a living by selling their handicrafts in North America. This employment helps craftspeople provide food, shelter, education, and health care for their families. SELFHELP Crafts of the World is one of the many programs of the Mennonite Central Committee, the relief and service agency of North American Mennonite and Brethren in Christ churches. SELFHELP has been helping disadvantaged craftspeople for more than forty-five years. For a catalogue, write to: SELFHELP Crafts of the World, 704 Main Street, Box 500, Akron, PA 17501; or call (717) 859-4971.

United Nations Children's Fund (UNICEF)

UNICEF concerns itself with the essential needs and problems of children, primarily those in developing countries. It helps plan and assist child care programs that are the responsibility of individual countries themselves. It is the policy of UNICEF to help children of both sides in an international conflict.

You are undoubtedly familiar with UNICEF Christmas cards. Each year UNICEF sells over a hundred million cards in more than a hundred countries, providing it with annual revenue of about $15 million. But you may not be aware that UNICEF also markets toys, books, games, calendars, and year round greeting cards. These gifts are designed to acquaint people with cultures around the world, and the profits go to help children all over the earth. To find the location of the UNICEF outlet closest to you, look up U.S. Committee for UNICEF in your phone book or call (800) FOR-KIDS. For a card and gift catalogue, write to The Winter Collection, U.S. Committee for UNICEF, 333 East 38th Street, New York, NY 10016; or call (212) 686-5522.

Pueblo to People

Pueblo to People is a nonprofit organization located in Houston, Texas, which was founded in 1979. This organization focuses its efforts on craft and agricultural cooperatives of very low-income people in Latin America. It works at the grass roots level, supporting organizations of the poor. Your purchases of its products not only provide people in Latin America with badly needed income, but give them a chance to learn organizational skills and democratic methods often taken for granted by more sophisticated societies.

Since its inception, Pueblo to People has paid over $4 million to craft and food producers in Latin America. Of each sales dollar, forty to forty-five cents goes directly to the producers; the rest goes to pay for operational expenses. For a catalogue, call (800) 843-5257 twenty-four hours a day. Featured items include handmade rugs, baskets, hand-blown glass, hand-loomed cloth, and ethnic clothing.

Alternative Christmas Activities for Churches

Over the years, we have kept a list of ideas that churches around the country have come up with to make their church programming more consistent with the spiritual meaning of Christmas. Scan the following list for ideas that your church might adapt, or use the list to stimulate your own brainstorming.

Ideas to reach out to other people

✳ Have a "Living, Giving Tree." Encourage families within the church to give a gift for the needy. Place the wrapped present under a living Christmas tree in a prominent place in the church.

✳ Begin the Christmas season with an undecorated Christmas tree. Each family that does an act that expresses the Christmas spirit is entitled to bring an ornament to put on the tree. At the end of the season the brightly decorated tree will be a testament to the community's goodwill toward others.

✳ Have someone make a large poster of the Christmas Pledge (see page 13) and tack it in a central location in the church. Leave room on it for church members to sign.

✳ As a church community, adopt a needy family.

✳ Have each willing member of the congregation choose a "secret friend," some friend or acquaintance to help out in some manner at some time during the holiday season. For example, help clean the house of an older person in anticipation of holiday visits.

* Put special ornaments on the church Christmas tree with the names of the people in the congregation who are sick, housebound, or in a nursing home, and could use a friendly visit or help with holiday chores.

Ideas to unite the church community

* Have a single-parent greens-gathering party.

* Have children interview their grandparents for stories of Christmas long ago. Print the stories in a special church newsletter.

* Have a "Fathers-and-Children Wrapping Session." Ask all the fathers and their children to bring family presents and wrapping paper to a special gathering. This will not only help out their wives but bring the men and their children closer together.

* Start a special campaign to visit church members who are in nursing homes and hospitals.

* Choose people to help with Christmas programming who can use more social interaction, rather than those who are already overcommitted.

Ideas to reduce commercialism

* Exchange gifts on St. Nicholas's Day (December 6) rather than Christmas Eve or Christmas Day, to save the true holiday for religious expression.

* Pledge not to exchange Christmas gifts with people within the congregation. Donate this money to a worthwhile cause.

* Have a church Christmas card for everyone to sign. As a symbolic statement that the earth's resources should be preserved, do not exchange cards with people within the congregation.

* Cut Christmas expenditures by 10 percent.

* Have a "Santa's Workshop." Each family donates a small gift or homemade present to a special children's bazaar. Each child brings a small amount of money and buys presents for other people in the family. (Gifts may be fifty cents apiece, for example.) The money goes to the church or some other worthwhile cause. This gives children the privilege of giving and keeps their presents to family members a secret.

* Pledge to reduce your children's television viewing during the holiday season and replace those hours with family activities.

Organize a discussion of commercialism versus the spirit of Christmas in the Sunday school.

✳ As a congregation, pledge to shop at those stores that delay their Christmas decorating until after Thanksgiving.

✳ Have an alternative Christmas tree that members can decorate with written ideas for a simpler Christmas.

✳ Make a banner that says TAKE TIME or KEEP IT SIMPLE and hang it in the church foyer.

✳ Each week of Advent, church bulletins could offer practical suggestions for carrying out each of the five ideas of the Christmas Pledge.

Ideas for church programming

✳ Sponsor an Unplug the Christmas Machine group workshop, the one on which this book is based. Through this workshop your church will help its members create more rewarding, more spiritual, and less stressful celebrations. People who participate in the workshop will go through many of the key exercises in this book, but they will have the added benefit of being able to function as a built-in support group for each other during the holiday season. The workshop can also serve as an outreach tool to acquaint people with your church community. Many church groups who have purchased the *Leader's Guide* in the past continue to give the workshop year after year.

The workshop is flexible and can be given in a four-hour block, a condensed two- or three-hour version, or as a series of one-hour segments to fit in with your adult education program. (Instructions on how to adapt the workshop are included in the guide.) The guide contains detailed instructions for conducting the workshop as well as a copy of a Participant's Manual to be photocopied for each participant.

For many years we published the *Leader's Guide to the Unplug the Christmas Machine* ourselves and sold it for $35.00. In conjunction with the revised edition of this book, the guide is now being published by William Morrow at a reduced price of $20.00. We apologize to those of you who tried to order the guide in recent years and couldn't reach us because of the out-of-date mailing address in earlier printings. Now you can simply order the guide from the publisher (see page 195) or through your local bookstore. We advise that you order it as early in the year as possible so you can do some advance planning.

❋ Offer a Christmas planning workshop to the congregation in early fall. The purpose of the workshop is to explore the church's role in the celebration. The session could follow this format:

1 List the church's traditional Christmas activities and consider these questions: Who is responsible for planning and carrying each one out? Who is each of the programs designed to benefit? Which work well?

2 What should the church's goals be at Christmas? Take some time to dream about creative ways the church could be a more positive force in restoring the meaning of the celebration. How well do your current holiday activities further your goals?

3 Formulate specific ways to reach these goals. You may wish to take these questions into consideration: How can the work involved in these activities be redistributed to relieve hardworking church members and include new, lonely, or single people? How can ongoing church responsibilities be reduced so that church leaders can spend more time with their families? How can church sermons and education classes reinforce the ideas generated in this planning session?

Making a Christmas budget

In an ideal world, people wouldn't have to think about money at Christmas. Adults could go through the holiday season as carefree as children and with no awareness of how the celebration translated into dollars and cents. Unfortunately, many adults not only have to think about money at Christmas, but worry about it as well. They worry about whether they have enough money to travel to see their relatives. They wonder if they can afford to buy their children the gifts they really want. And they find that they have to cut back on many of their holiday plans so that there will be enough money left over for everyday expenses.

But despite this worrying and economizing, many families still end up spending more money at Christmas than they can comfortably afford. We have found that setting up a holiday budget is a good way to keep your Christmas expenses under control. The first step in this process is to get a realistic picture of how you have been spending money in the past. Most people greatly underestimate how much money they spend at Christmas because there are scores of common but hidden holiday expenses. People not only spend money for obvious things like gifts, holiday food, and decorations, but also pay for a lot of "incidentals."

On the following pages you will find a list of typical holiday purchases. Take a few moments to place a check mark by each of the items you spent money on last year. No one family would have all of these expenses, but most people have more of them than they realize.

Gifts

✳ Store-bought gifts
✳ Craft supplies to make gifts
✳ Wrapping paper
✳ Tissue paper
✳ Ribbon
✳ Bows
✳ Professional gift wrapping
✳ Gift tags
✳ Brown paper for mailing

✳ Gift boxes
✳ Strapping tape
✳ Transparent tape
✳ Mailing costs
✳ Transportation for shopping
✳ Catalogues
✳ Other

Food

✳ Special kitchen equipment (plum pudding molds, Christmas cookie cutters, etc.)
✳ Baking ingredients (candied fruits, dates, nuts, butter, liquor, etc.)
✳ More convenience foods and restaurant meals because of busier schedules
✳ Extra food for holiday guests and parties

✳ Christmas Eve food ingredients
✳ Christmas dinner ingredients
✳ New Year's dinner ingredients
✳ Liquor
✳ Special holiday for your family (eggnog, fresh fruit baskets, nuts, etc.)

Entertaining

✳ Professional housecleaning
✳ Professional rug cleaning
✳ Professional yard work
✳ Catering
✳ Home repairs and modeling
✳ Invitations
✳ Extra cleaning products
✳ Extra glasses, plates, silver, serving dishes, table linens

✳ Flowers
✳ Candles
✳ Other special decorations
✳ Party clothes
✳ Dry cleaning
✳ New furniture
✳ New houseplants

Houseguests

* New linens (towels, sheets, pillowcases)
* Pillows, blankets
* Higher utility bills
* Home repairs
* Entertainment (movies, dinners out, museums, concerts)
* Extra transportation costs
* Toys and games for visiting children

Travel

* Cost of transportation (airfare, train tickets, gasoline, etc.)
* Car rental once you reach your destination
* Lodging
* Meals out
* Souvenirs
* Guidebooks
* Maps
* House gifts
* Games and toys for children while traveling
* Books and magazines for adults
* Disposable diapers
* Pet boarding
* Timed lights and burglar alarms for your house
* Travel insurance
* Luggage
* Car maintenance, supplies (chains, etc.), and repairs

Decorations

* Christmas tree
* Tree stand
* Lights
* Replacement bulbs
* Tree ornaments
* Outdoor wreath or wreath supplies
* Crèche
* Advent wreath
* Candles
* Other inside decorations
* Craft books and magazines
* Craft supplies
* Greens, cones, etc.
* Outdoor decorations

Christmas Cards

* The cards themselves
* Postage
* Photographs
* Copying or printing costs

Charity

✳ Increased church donations

✳ Donations to charity

✳ Other

Miscellaneous

✳ Long-distance phone calls

✳ Increased entertainment costs

✳ Film and camera supplies

✳ Camera

✳ Film developing

✳ New clothes and shoes

✳ Dry cleaning

✳ Haircuts

✳ Baby-sitting

✳ Wood for the fire

✳ Holiday tipping

✳ Christmas records, sheet music, or tapes

✳ Other

The next step in creating a holiday budget is to set a spending ceiling. (If you are married, involve your spouse in this decision.) Be realistic. Think about how much you spent last year and make any adjustments you feel are desirable.

SPENDING CEILING

Next, make some rough estimates of how you would like this money allocated and enter those figures in the following categories (don't worry about being too precise; these are only general indicators):

Food: $

Gifts: $

Entertaining guests: $

Travel: $

Charity: $

Family entertainment: $

Decorations: $

Miscellaneous: $

Finally, throughout the season, use the expense log that follows to keep a running tally of all your extra holiday expenses. From time to time, total up the various categories and compare your estimates with the actual figures. Then change your spending pattern if you see the need.

ACTUAL EXPENSE LOG

Date	Item	Category	Cost	Running total

Order Form for
The Leader's Guide to the
Unplug the Christmas Machine Workshop

The Unplug the Christmas Machine workshop helps participants create more rewarding, more spiritual, and less stressful celebrations. The *Leader's Guide* contains detailed instructions for conducting the workshop as well as a copy of the Participant's Manual to be photocopied for each participant.

Please return this form to the address below with your *check or money order* for $20.00 (the cost of the book) + $3.00 (shipping and handling) + appropriate state sales tax (or include tax exempt/ resale number here _____).

Make the check payable to William Morrow and Co. Allow four weeks for delivery.

Enclosed is a check for $_____ to bill to a/c 99110.

Name: _____

Shipping address: _____

(Street address) _____

_____

Phone: (_____) _____ Date of Order: _____

Mail to: William Morrow and Company, Inc.
                  Special Sales
                  1350 Avenue of the Americas,
                  New York, NY 10019
                  1–800–821–1513

Please note: *Price and availability are subject to change.*

ABOUT THE AUTHORS

Jo Robinson is a free-lance writer specializing in books about personal and social change. She is the co-author of four other books, including *Emotional Incest,* and the best-selling *Getting the Love You Want.* She lives in Portland, Oregon, with her husband and son.

Jean Coppock Staeheli continues to help people make changes in their lives through her work in the Portland Health Institute's clinical programs, graduate courses and workshops, and services to health professionals. She also writes about health related topics. Jean lives in Tigard, Oregon, with her husband and two daughters.